Narrative Frontiers

Essays at the Edge of Medicine and the Multiverse

Arthur Lazarus, MD, MBA

Narrative Frontiers

Essays at the Edge of Medicine and the Multiverse

Arthur Lazarus, MD, MBA

Academica Press
Washington

Library of Congress Cataloging-in-Publication Data
Names: Lazarus, Arthur L. (author)
Title: Narrative frontiers : essays at the edge of medicine and the multiverse | Lazarus, Arthur L.
Description: Washington : Academica Press, 2025. | Includes references.
Identifiers: LCCN 2025939419 | ISBN 9781680534047 (hardcover) | 9781680534054 (e-book)

ALSO BY ARTHUR LAZARUS

Neuroleptic Malignant Syndrome and Related Conditions (co-author)

Controversies in Managed Mental Health Care

Career Pathways in Psychiatry: Transition in Changing Times

MD/MBA: Physicians on the New Frontier of Medical Management

Every Story Counts: Exploring Contemporary Practice Through Narrative Medicine

Medicine on Fire: A Narrative Travelogue

Narrative Medicine: The Fifth Vital Sign

Narrative Medicine: Harnessing the Power of Storytelling through Essays

Story Treasures: Medical Essays and Insights in the Narrative Tradition

21st Century Schizoid Health Care: Essays and Reflections to Keep You Sane on Your Medical Travels

Narrative Medicine: New and Selected Essays

Narrative Rx: A Quick Guide to Narrative Medicine for Students, Residents, and Attendings

For curious and compassionate caregivers
advancing the frontiers of medicine.

Contents

“Somewhere, something incredible is waiting to be known.”
— Carl Sagan

Preface

Why title this book *Narrative Frontiers: Essays at the Edge of Medicine and the Multiverse?*

The title reflects the spirit of exploration that underpins this collection of essays. Medicine, at its core, is a field of boundaries – between life and death, science and art, the known and the unknown. Yet, as these essays reveal, medicine also exists on a frontier, where human stories and cutting-edge advancements converge in unexpected ways.

The word “narrative” serves as a reminder that at the heart of medicine lies storytelling: the stories of patients, the reflections of caregivers, and the ever-evolving tale of health care itself. Through narrative, we make sense of the mysteries of illness and healing. Stories are the threads that connect science to humanity, grounding the cold precision of data in the warmth of shared experience.

“Frontiers” suggests a place of discovery and challenge, a terrain where innovation pushes boundaries. Today’s frontiers in medicine are not just physical or scientific; they extend into the conceptual realms of artificial intelligence (AI), bioethics, societal change, and even speculative ideas that belong more to science fiction than to the clinic – at least for now.

And then there’s the “multiverse.” While it nods to science fiction, the term also symbolizes the vast and overlapping worlds that shape modern medicine. Each essay in this collection touches on one of these worlds – whether it’s the universe of a patient’s unique perspective, the realities of global health disparities, or the speculative futures envisioned by advancements in technology. The multiverse evokes a sense of limitless possibility, a reminder that medicine is not confined to a single narrative or pathway.

This title, then, encapsulates the scope and ambition of these essays: to explore the intersection of medicine with broader societal forces, to navigate the edges of what we know, and to imagine what might lie beyond.

As you turn the pages of *Narrative Frontiers,* you will find essays that challenge, inspire, and provoke reflection. They explore medicine not just as a profession or science but as a human endeavor, shaped by the stories we tell and the innovations we pursue. From the ethical dilemmas of artificial intelligence to the personal struggles of burnout and fortitude, from the futuristic landscapes of AI-guided treatment to the deeply rooted traditions of care, this collection seeks to bridge the familiar and the extraordinary.

My hope is that these essays will offer more than just information or insight; they will offer a lens through which to see medicine anew. Whether you are a physician, a patient, or someone simply curious about the threads connecting health care to our rapidly changing world, this book invites you to journey to the edges of what we know – and to fancy what could be.

Welcome to the new – narrative – frontier.

Prologue

1.

The New Frontier in American Medicine

Surgery is often considered a "frontier" medical specialty – and with robotics and newer AI-assisted technologies, it still is. But just 10 years ago, who would have guessed that some surgeons – bariatric specialists, in particular – would be losing their jobs to the weight-loss glucagon-like-peptide-1 receptor agonist (GLP-1) class of medications?

Research published in *JAMA Network Open* in October 2024 found a 25.6% decrease in bariatric surgery procedures in non-diabetic patients with obesity between the last 6 months of 2022 versus the last 6 months of 2023, but a 132.6% increase in patients prescribed GLP-1 drugs. That means some surgeons – and programs and facilities that cater to weigh reduction management – will be going out of business and closing.

Coincident with this trend, many bariatric surgeons are frequently checking their specialty's job boards for new or alternative jobs. Some are enrolling in refresher courses for other kinds of foregut surgery, such as hernia repair, gallbladder removal, or esophageal procedures. Other surgeons are pivoting to telehealth. However, it is quite possible for business to pick up given the apparent greater efficacy of bariatric surgery versus medication: GLP-1 agonists can achieve about 14% total body weight loss; surgery is approximately 30% after a year to 18 months, according to a 2022 review article published in *Advances in Therapy*. Estimates vary, however.

Also, the comparison between drugs and surgery is confounded by long-term outcomes. GLP-1 agonists may have intolerable side effects and rebound weight gain. Bariatric surgery may be irreversible, and surgery-related complications may occur early and late. Published head-to-head comparisons are rare. It is likely that when the pendulum stops swinging, there will be an uptick in surgical cases again. Just as cancer treatment often requires a combination of surgery and drugs, combination therapy will be the treatment plan for many patients with obesity. But no one can predict the future with certainty.

Which brings us back to the "new" frontier. Wayne Gretzky, considered the greatest ice hockey player of all time, had the ability to predict where the puck will be, which is how he scored so many goals. Nostradamus had the ability to prophesize and predict future events. John F. Kennedy had the ability to stand on a "frontier of unknown opportunities and perils, a frontier of unfilled hopes and threats," as he famously remarked in his 1960 presidential acceptance speech. Physicians must be prophets, too, as they stand on the new frontier of medicine. They must possess an ability to predict future trends in medicine if they desire to practice on the cutting edge.

Of course, many bariatric surgeons will adjust and perhaps diversify their surgical repertoire, alternating it with acute care surgery. However, the prospect of taking on general surgery – where often it's one-and-done – goes against the reason many bariatric surgeons chose weight-loss surgery as a specialty: to have longer-term relationships with their patients. I'm sure they'll find a way to reconfigure their practice – even their career – when bariatric demand has evened out. This will be their new frontier.

Medicine is constantly in flux. There will never be stabilization of all the phenomena and moving parts that comprise the profession and impact practice. The new frontier was Kennedy's way of communicating this challenge on a larger scale. "Can a nation organized and governed such as ours endure?" he asked, answering "That is the choice our nation must make – a choice…between the public interest and the private comfort, between national greatness and national decline…"

Despite the harsh ways I may characterize contemporary medical practice in the U.S. throughout this book, I remain optimistic. I do believe we can achieve a state of greatness and prevent its further decline. Do we really have a choice? JFK didn't think so. He was resolute in his belief that America will pave the way for the rest of the world: "All mankind waits upon our decision. A whole world looks to see what we will do. We cannot fail their trust. We cannot fail to try."

Eight years later, at the 1968 democratic national convention in Chicago, with JFK and his brother Bobby now gone, the whole world was indeed watching. And it has watched before – and since – then. America, and U.S. medicine, is the greatest ever known. Our system may be in disarray, but its strength, which rests on a foundation of research and technology, remains intact. I would even go so far as to say we are on the leading edge of a new frontier.

As we stand at this precipice, the challenge is not only to adapt but to innovate and lead. The frontier is not just about discovering new treatments or technologies; it is about redefining our approach to care, embracing holistic and personalized medicine, and ensuring equitable access for all. The future of medicine will be shaped by our willingness to embrace change and lead movements, to collaborate across disciplines, and to remain steadfast in our commitment to improving the human condition.

In this changing landscape, the role of the physician will also transform, as witnessed by our surgical colleagues. We must become not only healers but also pioneers and advocates for our patients in a world that is increasingly complex and interconnected. The narrative of medicine is one of constant reinvention, and as we write the next chapter, let us do so with courage, compassion, and a vision for a healthier, more equitable world.

This is the new frontier in medicine: a place where innovation meets empathy, where science and humanity converge, and where the possibilities are as vast and varied as the multiverse itself. Let us embrace it with open minds and hopeful hearts, ready to shape the future of health for generations to come.

Section 1:

The New Frontier

2.

Hospitals Are the New Coliseum

The enduring allure of violence as spectacle has spread from the arena to the football field to the hospital.

I recently attended a professional ice hockey game. The fans were mostly entertained by the fights that erupted between opposing players, especially if one drew blood. Several days later, I watched a professional football game on television. There were many violent collisions and a near-bench-clearing brawl. One player suffered a severe concussion accompanied by the "fencing response," requiring immediate on-field medical attention.

I began to tune out the game and think instead about how injuries sustained by professional athletes might mirror those suffered by gladiators. This comparison reveals a stark continuity in the human fascination with violence as entertainment, raising questions about the progress of civilization over centuries – have we evolved all that much since the Romans? Do we not still have an insatiable appetite for death and destruction?

The societal contexts and implications may have changed since ancient times, but football players (and other athletes) and gladiators endure significant physical risks to perform for the masses. Let's compare and contrast these two elite figures and see how they parallel modern-day patients in hospitals.

Gladiators: The Entertainment of Death

In ancient Rome, gladiators were warriors forced – or sometimes voluntarily agreeing – to fight to the death or until incapacitated for public viewing. These contests were brutal, often fatal, and underscored by a voyeuristic culture that glorified violence as both a sport and a tool for political control. The arena symbolized power, reinforcing the dominance of the privileged who orchestrated these events for the "bread and circuses" of the populace.

While gladiators sometimes achieved celebrity status, their lives were expendable. Injuries, infections, or death were common, yet the crowd's appetite for violence fueled the demand. The gladiators' plight exemplifies a societal desensitization to human suffering when framed as an exhibition.

Football Players: The New Gladiators

American football, while far less overtly deadly, retains echoes of this gladiatorial culture. Athletes, celebrated as heroes, sacrifice their bodies for entertainment and economic opportunity. Traumatic injuries, including concussions and chronic traumatic encephalopathy (CTE), reveal the sport's hidden toll. CTE, caused by repetitive head trauma – now seen in virtually all contact sports – leads to progressive brain degeneration, with symptoms including memory loss, aggression, depression, and even suicide.

Despite increased awareness, the allure of high-impact plays – the "big hits" – continues to draw millions of fans. The violence is sanitized, regulated by rules and protective equipment, but the underlying dynamic remains: players suffer, and the crowd cheers. Worse still, the show has filtered down to college and high school athletics, where unprecedented numbers of injuries occur, and where young athletes – desperate for a chance at fame in their name, image, and likeness – accept the risks with little real understanding of the consequences.

Patients: The Modern-Day Warriors

This pattern is eerily familiar to those of us who have worked in hospitals, where the vulnerable, sick, or injured are often further harmed and become pawns in a system designed to extract profits. Whether on the field or in a hospital bed, patients' agony becomes a form of currency. Hospital and insurance executives, bloodthirsty for revenue, turn suffering into a form of spectacle, albeit one obscured by layers of corporate jargon and bureaucratic policies. In this system, a patient's pain is less important than their billing codes. Just as athletes are celebrated while their injuries are quietly swept aside, patients are reduced to cases, numbers, or "problems to solve" – a depersonalization that hides the human cost of care.

Doctors: Collateral Damage

The transformation of hospitals into coliseums not only exploits patients but also inflicts collateral damage on doctors. Physicians, like players on the field, are expected to perform under immense pressure, often at the expense of their own well-being. Administrative burdens, unrealistic productivity metrics, and moral injury from witnessing preventable suffering have created a crisis of burnout and despair. In many ways, doctors become spectators in their own arena, forced to watch as bureaucratic systems override their training and instincts. Stripped of their agency, they too are reduced to cogs in a machine that values efficiency over empathy, profit over healing. While patients may represent the fallen gladiators, doctors find themselves in the precarious role of reluctant participants, caught between their desire to care and the constraints of a system indifferent to their humanity.

Parallels and Divergences

Both gladiatorial games and professional football thrive on public fascination with physical dominance and violence. Spectators detach themselves from the human loss, focusing instead on the drama of the game. Participants – whether athletes or patients – are frequently viewed as symbols or performers rather than individuals with vulnerabilities. This makes it easier for audiences, administrators, and executives to turn a blind eye and ignore the toll these systems exact on people's lives.

The issue of agency highlights key differences among groups. Modern football players, on the surface, choose to compete, often driven by passion for the sport or the promise of financial reward. Gladiators, by contrast, were frequently enslaved or coerced into the arena, denied their autonomy. Yet "choice" in football is complicated by outside pressures, such as poverty and limited career options, much like patients "choosing" care options under a fragmented healthcare system. For many, options are determined less by preference than by circumstance.

Advancements in medical knowledge offer another point of comparison. In contemporary sports, injuries and their long-term consequences – like CTE – are better understood than in gladiatorial times. Yet changes to prioritize athlete safety remain slow, as profits often take precedence. Similarly, modern medicine has unparalleled technology, research, and treatment capabilities, yet systemic reform to prioritize patient care over profits has stalled. The gladiators had no protections, but how far have we come when hospitals are designed more like coliseums, ruled by executive elites watching the action from above?

Has Civilization Evolved?

In some ways, yes – human rights, medical ethics, and safety standards have progressed. The gladiatorial arena is no longer a literal killing field. However, our ongoing fascination with violence as entertainment, coupled with the exploitation of human suffering in modern systems, shows that certain elements of human nature remain unchanged. In sports, as in health care, the transformation is more aesthetic than fundamental. Players still fall to cheers and applause, and patients suffer unseen while profits quietly roll in and line executives' pockets.

The challenge lies in harmonizing the tensions between progress and exploitation and between spectacle and ethics. Can society evolve beyond the need for violence as entertainment, whether on the field or within the walls of a hospital? Can we dismantle the systems that commodify suffering – be it an athlete's sacrifice or a patient's illness – in the name of profit and power? Or will we continue to justify these systems as tradition, culture, or necessity? These questions remain as relevant today as they were centuries ago.

To balance these tensions, executives must learn what doctors, patients, and world-class athletes already understand: that the relentless pursuit of performance, whether in the hospital or on the gridiron, demands not only pushing limits but also preserving the strength and humanity of those involved. Failing to do so ensures they remain complicit in the very system that consumes everyone within it.

3.

The Intersection of Economic Systems and Mental Health

Reclaiming holistic psychiatry through the biopsychosocial lens.

A colleague, a clinical psychologist, read the preceding essay and commented, "People are becoming more cynical because the American Dream for so many is now out of reach. This is what happens when you have savage capitalism: capitalism devoid of values and morality where nothing is ever enough."

My friend touched on a significant issue that many have observed in contemporary society. When capitalism becomes unmoored from ethical considerations, it can create a culture of relentless competition, exploitation, and inequality. The ideals of the American Dream—opportunity, upward mobility, and fairness – become unattainable for large segments of the population. Instead, we see escalating economic disparity, the erosion of social safety nets, and a pervasive sense of disillusionment.

Cynicism often arises when people feel powerless to change systems they perceive as unjust. Savage capitalism, as he described it, prioritizes profit over people, stripping away the shared values and sense of community that once underpinned the American Dream. Without those, it's easy to see why people might become skeptical or distrustful of institutions that no longer seem to serve them.

My colleague heads a group of mental health clinicians specializing in the treatment of individuals, couples, and families experiencing anxiety, stress, depression, trauma, and many more difficulties. In his view, "savage capitalism" – more than ever – contributes to a host of psychological disorders. This system fosters a relentless pursuit of material success, exacerbating feelings of inadequacy, hopelessness, and alienation among those who struggle to meet its often unattainable demands.

Based on previous discussions with my colleague, I know that from his perspective, capitalism without values breeds a culture where people are valued more for their productivity than their humanity, leading to widespread burnout, fractured relationships, and a loss of purpose. Such a context undermines mental health, intensifying the very conditions – stress, inequality, and isolation – that our patients seek help to navigate.

Economic systems are not merely abstract forces but deeply interwoven with the psychological and emotional fabric of society, shaping both collective and personal well-being. When an economic system such as "savage capitalism" prioritizes profits over people, it can lead to job insecurity or unaffordable housing or health care. These material conditions create chronic stress, which is a significant contributor to mental health issues like anxiety, depression, and trauma.

Moreover, economic systems shape societal values. In a system driven by relentless competition and consumerism, individuals may internalize the belief that their worth is tied to productivity or material success. This mindset can erode self-esteem, foster social isolation, and increase the prevalence of burnout. On a societal level, such systems can weaken community ties, amplify divisions, and fuel a sense of collective despair – all of which feed into the growing cynicism and mental health crises seen today.

Understanding this interconnection is vital for clinicians, policymakers, and community leaders. Addressing mental health challenges requires not just individual treatment but also widespread change to create an environment that fosters psychological resilience and emotional well-being.

Psychiatrists, with their deep training in the biological sciences, are uniquely positioned to understand the complex interplay between biological, psychological, and social factors in mental health. However, there is growing concern that the emphasis on biological treatments—such as psychopharmacology – has led some practitioners to underemphasize the impact of economic and psychosocial stressors.

For example, while medications can be highly effective for managing symptoms, they do not address root causes such as financial insecurity, workplace stress, or social determinants of health that may underlie a patient's mental health struggles. Failing to integrate these dimensions into care risks providing incomplete treatment, where symptoms are managed without addressing the broader context of an individual's life.

Psychiatrists can benefit from embracing a more holistic approach to mental health care, one that integrates the biological, psychological, and social dimensions of well-being. By rebalancing their approach to encompass these dimensions, psychiatrists can offer more effective and compassionate care that recognizes the interconnected nature of mental health and society.

George Engel, MD, espoused this concept many decades ago. It's disappointing that it has not rooted in contemporary psychiatric practice, where psychiatrists handle the medication and non-medical therapists conduct psychotherapy.

Engel's biopsychosocial model, which he proposed in the late 1970s as a revolutionary framework for understanding health and illness, emphasized that health cannot be fully understood through a purely biological lens but must account for psychological and social dimensions as well. His work remains a cornerstone of medical theory, yet, its application in modern psychiatric practice often falls short.

The fragmentation – psychiatrists focusing almost exclusively on medication while psychotherapy is left to non-medical therapists – illustrates a troubling drift from Engel's vision. This division of labor can result in a narrowed scope of care, where psychiatrists are seen as pharmacologists rather than holistic practitioners addressing the full spectrum of a patient's needs. While the collaboration between psychiatrists and therapists can be effective, it risks compartmentalizing care if the two sides fail to integrate their approaches.

In fact, fewer than half of psychiatrists today conduct psychotherapy. Their failure to fully embrace Engel's model may stem from the greater influence by the biomedical model, driven in part by advances in neurobiology and pharmacology, as well as economic factors like insurance reimbursements that favor brief medication management visits over extended psychotherapy sessions. This shift may inadvertently reinforce the notion that mental health is primarily a biological issue, sidelining the psychosocial elements that Engel viewed as equally critical.

To address this, psychiatry needs a cultural shift that reclaims the biopsychosocial model as central to its practice. Psychiatrists can benefit from re-engaging with psychotherapy as a vital skill set, integrating it into their work rather than delegating it entirely. Additionally, medical education and continuing professional development should emphasize the importance of viewing patients through Engel's holistic lens. By reinvigorating the biopsychosocial model in psychiatry, the field can move toward more comprehensive care that recognizes the full complexity of human mental health, including the economic forces driving mental health outcomes.

4.

Navigating Health Care with Grace and Determination

Practice the art of "respectful relentlessness" to satisfy your healthcare needs.

I'm relatively new to Medicare. I know it's not perfect as far as insurance goes, nor is it free, as many people believe. Oh, sure, you can sign up for one of those bargain-basement Medicare "Advantage" plans and pay nothing or next to nothing – but as the adage goes: you get what you pay for.

Medicare Advantage Plans: Benefits and Drawbacks

Medicare Advantage plans, also known as Medicare Part C, are often promoted as a cost-effective alternative to traditional Medicare. These plans typically offer lower premiums and may include additional benefits, such as vision, dental, or hearing coverage, that traditional Medicare does not. However, these lower upfront costs can come with trade-offs that affect flexibility and access to care.

One major limitation is that Medicare Advantage plans are generally not as portable as traditional Medicare. Most plans operate within a specific network of doctors, hospitals, and other providers, which can make accessing care outside the plan's service area challenging, particularly for those who travel frequently or live in multiple locations (I'm guilty on both counts). Additionally, these plans often require a higher degree of preauthorization for services, meaning that patients may need approval from the insurer before undergoing certain treatments, procedures, or tests. This can delay care and add administrative complexity, neither of which is desirable in an elderly population.

Another concern relates to the overall quality of care. While some Medicare Advantage plans perform well in terms of patient satisfaction and outcomes, others have been criticized for their limitations on access to care and for sometimes denying necessary services, cherry-picking certain procedures and targeting them for cost-reduction. The variability in quality can make it essential for individuals to thoroughly research and compare plans before enrolling.

For individuals who prioritize flexibility and access to a broad range of providers, traditional Medicare, often supplemented with a "Medigap" policy and a separate (Part D) plan for prescription drug coverage, may be a better choice despite the higher premiums. Understanding the differences between traditional Medicare and Medicare Advantage is critical to making an informed decision based on personal health needs and circumstances.

I chose traditional Medicare and felt informed. I went to my primary care doctor's office for my annual wellness exam. I left very frustrated. First, I was told by someone in the front-office that any current symptoms I wished to discuss might be an extra charge. What?

Next, I was interviewed extensively by a semi-retired nurse, who asked me a battery of questions more appropriate for a person incapable of living independently.

I was most annoyed, however, that my doctor never physically examined me.

What kind of check-up is this?

Medicare Annual Wellness Visit vs. Annual Physical Exam

I discovered that there is a difference between Medicare's Annual Wellness Visit (AWV) and a standard annual physical exam: the difference lies in their purpose, coverage, and what they include. The AWV, covered by Medicare Part B at no cost to the patient (if the provider accepts Medicare), focuses on preventive care and health management. It involves a health risk assessment, a review of medical and family history, and a discussion of current medications.

The visit also includes cognitive impairment screening (hence, the clock drawing test), the creation or updating of a personalized preventive services plan, and recommendations for preventive measures like screenings or vaccinations. Patients may also discuss advance care planning during this visit. However, the AWV does not include a hands-on physical exam or the evaluation of existing health problems (hence, the reason for the additional cost).

In contrast, a standard annual physical exam is a comprehensive assessment of overall health, often covered only by private insurance, Medigap, or Medicare Advantage plans. This visit includes a thorough physical examination, such as listening to the heart and lungs or palpating the abdomen. It may also involve diagnostic tests, addressing symptoms, or managing chronic conditions. The focus of an annual physical is more diagnostic and current health-focused, rather than preventive and forward-looking like the AWV.

If you are on Medicare, it is essential to understand these distinctions to avoid unexpected charges, particularly if you are expecting one type of visit and receive another, as was my case. Medicare can be just as complicated as private insurance, which is inexcusable considering the higher degree of cognitive challenges in the population it serves.

In fact, to sign in to my Medicare account using my online Social Security account, I am required to memorize and enter an 8-digit number sent to my iPhone. An 8-digit number falls within the upper limit of the typical digit span capacity, indicating that while many individuals can recall such a sequence immediately, it may be beyond the average short-term memory capabilities of many older adults. Need I say more?

Well, yes, which leads me to the last section about the relentless pursuit of your healthcare needs.

Respectful Relentlessness

In the beginning of this book, I addressed a fundamental truth: Americans across all age groups – not just those eligible for Medicare – are furious over the state of health care. Until meaningful reform is achieved, the best advice I can offer for ensuring your medical needs are met is to adopt a mindset of "respectful relentlessness." This approach involves advocating firmly for yourself or a loved one while demonstrating genuine respect for the expertise, challenges, and constraints faced by healthcare providers.

Here are some actionable tips to practice respectful relentlessness:

- ☐ **State your expectations directly.** For example, when advocating for a timely appointment, you might say, "My specialists have informed me that it is medically important that I am seen in your office within the next few weeks." If you are placed on a waitlist, follow up regularly to check the status, even if the office does not contact you first.
- ☐ **Prioritize respectful conversation over confrontation.** Use empathetic phrasing like, "I know you are very busy..." while staying focused on the goal: your health. Avoid getting drawn into negativity, which only detracts from achieving the care you need.
- ☐ **Encourage direct communication between clinicians.** When usual channels fail, request that your doctors speak directly to one another to clarify the urgency or priority of your situation. Physicians are often juggling multiple demands, and your persistence in fostering communication can profoundly impact your care – or that of a loved one.
- ☐ **Keep Detailed Records:** Maintain a file of your medical history, test results, medications, and correspondence with healthcare providers. Being organized and having this information readily available demonstrates responsibility and helps expedite decisions.
- ☐ **Bring an Advocate:** If you feel overwhelmed or unsure how to navigate a situation, bring a trusted family member or friend to appointments. They can provide support, take notes, and help advocate for your needs.
- ☐ **Ask Clarifying Questions:** If you don't understand something a provider says, don't hesitate to ask for clarification. Phrasing like, "Could you explain that in simpler terms?" or "Can you help me understand how this fits with what I've been told previously?" shows engagement without confrontation.
- ☐ **Research Your Options:** While respecting your provider's expertise, take the initiative to educate yourself about your

condition and available treatments. This allows you to engage in informed discussions and ask specific questions that can guide decisions.

- **Use Online Portals:** Take advantage of patient portals to send messages, request prescription refills, or check test results. These platforms offer a documented, direct line of communication and can save time for both you and your provider.
- **Be Prepared for Appointments:** Examinations can cause anxiety which can cause us to be forgetful. Write down your questions, symptoms, and priorities ahead of time. This helps ensure that all your concerns are addressed efficiently during the limited time you have with your provider.
- **Acknowledge Positive Efforts:** When a healthcare professional goes out of their way to help you, express genuine gratitude. A simple "Thank you for taking the time to address my concern" fosters goodwill and encourages further engagement.
- **Escalate When Necessary:** If you encounter roadblocks, politely but firmly request to speak with a supervisor or patient advocate. Many healthcare systems have ombudsmen or other resources to help resolve issues.

In a healthcare landscape fraught with hurdles and barriers, respectful relentlessness can be a powerful tool to navigate the challenges and ensure your voice is heard.

5.

Arriving on the Medical Scene

Achieving milestones in a landscape of independent paths.

Writers and musicians increasingly are turning to independent publishing and recording to disseminate their works. Wayne Whittaker, a Los Angeles-based multi-instrumentalist, singer-songwriter, producer, and the man behind the rock group Pigeon Club, knows a thing or two about indie music making, having recorded albums yet consigned to spending "Another Year in the Minors," the title of Pigeon Club's 2024 release.

The title of the album says it all: the process of grinding it out, the notion of self-belief, the idea that a break is just around the corner as long as you keep your nose to the grindstone and are somehow noticed by someone influential who can promote your talents.

"Another year in the minors. The disappointment designers…Maybe today will be the day."

Who knows?

When are you hoping to "break out?" What will your breakout day look like? Will you experience more than 15 minutes of fame? Do you even desire fame? What is your vision of "having arrived on the scene?"

The idea of "breaking out" and what that looks like varies greatly from person to person. For some, it's not about fame at all but about making a meaningful impact – whether by reaching the right audience, influencing a small but dedicated community, or creating something enduring. Fame, with all its trappings, is a goal for some but a burden for others. For many creatives, the true reward lies in the work itself and the fulfillment it brings.

If “breaking out” means finally being seen or acknowledged, your breakout day could be a moment when your work connects deeply with others – when you receive an unexpected note from someone whose life was changed by your words, music, or art. It might not look like a red carpet or a viral explosion but could instead be quiet, personal, and profoundly satisfying.

On the other hand, some creators envision “arriving on the scene” as attaining a platform large enough to amplify their voice. That might mean achieving bestseller status, playing to sold-out venues, or receiving recognition from industry peers. Even then, the process is ongoing. For many, the idea of "having arrived" is less a destination and more a milestone in an evolving journey.

Ultimately, whether or not one desires fame, the real vision should be centered on authenticity and purpose. What matters most is creating work that aligns with your values and that fulfills the reason you started creating in the first place. The “breakout moment” may come when you least expect it – or it might never come at all in the way you'd envisioned. The key is to keep moving forward, staying true to your craft, and defining success on your own terms.

My breakout moment came unexpectedly in my last year of residency. I over-ruled a surgical attending and ordered the transfer of his patient to the psychiatric inpatient unit. The patient was disfigured by head and neck surgery, which caused him to feel hopeless and attempt suicide. The surgeon opposed inpatient treatment believing it would stigmatize his patient. “He’s already stigmatized,” I told the surgeon as I raised my voice, standing toe-to-toe in hospital corridor. The surgeon acquiesced. The patient was transferred. I acted alone, never consulting my attending. As a result of the experience, I felt as though I had finally arrived.

That moment, standing toe-to-toe with the surgeon and holding my ground, represents more than a personal triumph. It reflects the enormous responsibility physicians bear – not just to treat illness but to see the person behind the diagnosis, to recognize suffering beyond the physical, and to advocate fiercely for those who cannot advocate for themselves.

My choice to act decisively, without consulting my attending, wasn’t just a step forward in my professional journey; it was a leap into the role of an independent and ethical leader. Sometimes, arriving on the scene isn't about conformity or approval but about taking a stand, trusting your instincts, and doing what's right, no matter the risk.

Moments like these define careers and set the stage for a lifetime of courageous, patient-centered practice. They often transcend the technical milestones of completing training or passing board exams. These events are marked by a shift in confidence, autonomy, and purpose – when the physician transitions from following to leading, from learning to teaching, or from practicing to advocating.

For medical students, the experience of performing their first solo history and physical exam, synthesizing findings, and presenting a coherent assessment and plan often signifies a breakthrough in their journey. Similarly, receiving heartfelt gratitude from a patient or family member after explaining a diagnosis or offering comfort reflects their growing ability to connect deeply and meaningfully.

Another pivotal moment can occur when a student challenges a teaching point during a lecture or on rounds, demonstrating the confidence and critical thinking that signal they are beginning to think like a physician. I had a few of those moments when I was the only person among my fellow students and senior residents who had the correct answer to clinical questions asked by probing attendings, a practice also known as "pimping" that is now frowned upon because it fosters a culture of humiliation and anxiety rather than one of constructive learning.

Nevertheless, confidently providing the correct answer, especially when others cannot, are significant milestones in a medical student's journey. They represent more than just knowledge—they highlight a student's preparedness, ability to think critically, synthesize information, and perform under pressure.

For residents, their defining moments might come during their first independent management of a critical situation, such as leading a code, where their actions earn the trust and respect of their team. Another significant milestone occurs when a resident makes a tough but ethical decision for a patient, prioritizing the patient's well-being over protocol or hierarchy, as in my example of transferring a patient to inpatient psychiatry despite opposition. Additionally, mentoring junior residents or medical students, and witnessing their growth and success as a result of that mentorship, highlights the residents' role as a leader and teacher.

For attending physicians, "arriving" often means taking on roles beyond patient care. This could involve advocating for organizational change, such as improving patient care policies or championing resident wellness programs, and seeing those efforts lead to tangible improvements. It might also involve being recognized by colleagues, patients, or the community as a trusted leader or expert in their field. For some, it's the development and implementation of innovative treatments, protocols, or teaching methods that have a measurable impact on outcomes or education.

A classmate one year my junior was considered a "sleeper" in medical school, only to "arrive" a few decades later. He became a world leader in the development and use of minimally invasive hip and knee replacements, and he holds several patents for their design. He has authored over 420 textbook chapters and research articles published in peer-reviewed journals. In addition to having lectured at hundreds of medical meetings around the world, he annually hosts numerous visiting national and international surgeons to observe his surgery and practice. I'd say he has "arrived."

Across all stages of medical training and practice, the moments that signify "arrival" often share universal themes. These include acts of advocacy, creativity, and ethical clarity – times when physicians step beyond technical proficiency into roles where they shape their environment, inspire trust, and make lasting impacts on individuals or systems. These defining events mark the transition from learning medicine to truly living it, embodying its ideals and responsibilities.

6.

From Breaking Point to Break Down

Physicians can turn moments of crisis
into opportunities for discovery and growth.

There is a huge difference between "breaking out," as I discussed in the preceding essay, and "breaking down," which is the consequence of a severe mental health struggle. Breakdowns in doctors manifest in various ways, and many show tremendous resilience before they reach their breaking point. Additionally, not all physicians who reach their breaking point have a breakdown. Let's sort this all out – breaking points and breakdowns – and give some examples.

Breaking points are thresholds – the moments when the weight of responsibility, exhaustion, or emotional toll becomes almost unbearable. These are not necessarily breakdowns but critical junctures that challenge a physician's endurance. For example, consider the resident working 80-hour weeks who, after losing multiple patients in quick succession, finds themselves questioning their ability to continue. They may not quit or collapse, but the breaking point forces them to reassess their coping strategies and support systems.

Breakdowns, on the other hand, occur when the cumulative stress surpasses what a person can manage, resulting in significant psychological distress or dysfunction. There is a physical, emotional, or psychological collapse that results from unrelenting pressure or other mental health challenges. This could manifest as severe depression, anxiety, substance use, or physical symptoms of an acute or chronic illness. Physicians are particularly susceptible due to the culture of medicine, which often discourages vulnerability and prioritizes endurance over self-care. An attending physician, for instance, might suffer a breakdown after years of silently battling burnout, triggered by an adverse patient outcome or a sudden personal crisis, e.g., divorce or family illness.

However, not every physician who reaches a breaking point experiences a breakdown. Some show tremendous resilience, finding ways to recalibrate and heal. For instance, a surgeon might channel their frustration and fatigue into advocacy, working to improve organizational issues contributing to burnout. Another might lean on peer support groups or therapy to process their experiences and regain equilibrium.

Examples abound of physicians navigating these challenges, with both positive and negative outcomes. The late Dr. Lorna Breen, an emergency medicine physician in New York City during the early days of the COVID-19 pandemic, tragically exemplifies how relentless stress can culminate in a breakdown with devastating consequences (she died by suicide). Family members founded the Dr. Lorna Breen Heroes Foundation in her honor to help advocate for a world where seeking mental health services is universally viewed as a sign of strength rather than weakness.

Dr William West, Jr, an ophthalmology resident, also took his life to the surprise of his family, co-residents and attendings. They never noticed anything "wrong," which is not unusual in physicians given their high degree of resiliency. Yet, the note he left behind painted a different picture. It read, in part: "To those in a position of authority over residents, a simple reminder that we come to you seeking the possibility of a better life. Some of us with challenges you do not see or backgrounds of which you are not aware ... I hope that an effort can be made to understand, support, and mentor the residents rather than simply to assess and drive them toward their highest potential as doctors." There were clearly aspects about Dr. West's training experience that he perceived as toxic.

Dr. Sarah DeParis, also an ophthalmologist, described a "Britney Spears moment" – a throwback to the pop star's nervous breakdown-induced shaved head in 2007. Chronic exhaustion and despair resulted in sudden "hysterical crying," triggering a moment of "scissor-wielding desperation." Despite seeking help for PTSD from years of chronic stress, Dr. DeParis felt it was in her best interest to leave practice (she is now the director of quality and clinical standards at the American Academy of Ophthalmology).

Conversely, Dr. Rana Awdish used her personal crisis as a catalyst for significant change and discovery. She is a critical care physician who experienced a life-threatening medical emergency when she suffered a major hemorrhage during her pregnancy. Her near-death experience and subsequent recovery led her to critically reassess the healthcare system from the perspective of a vulnerable patient and alter her approach to medicine and patient care, which she wrote about in her memoir *In Shock: My Journey from Death to Recovery and the Redemptive Power of Hope*.

Breaking points and breakdowns are part of the human experience, and physicians are no exception. Recognizing the signs and creating a culture that encourages support and recovery is critical to sustaining the profession. Addressing these challenges openly – through mentorship, peer support, and cultural reconfiguration – can help ensure that breaking points serve as opportunities for growth rather than paths to breakdowns.

I reached my breaking point in medical school, and I had a near-breakdown in my first year of residency. I've written extensively about both incidents. The events that caused them are not nearly as important as the methods I utilized to handle them. Without a doubt, professional help was the most important step – I would say a prerequisite for coping and recovery.

Sometimes it can be difficult to know where to draw the line between "suck it up and deal with it" and "get help before you break." Always err on the side of seeking help early by seeing a skilled psychiatrist or psychotherapist. Additionally, combining therapy with medication such as SSRIs may be necessary to treat major depression and trauma. It is well known that the cumulative stress of practicing medicine can be a traumatic experience and risk factor for PTSD.

There is no shame in seeking help; the stigma is lessening. Organizations are working to eliminate mental health language on credentialing and licensing applications and increase awareness of the need for physicians to seek care without retribution. Early intervention may prevent physicians from having regrets or afterthoughts, as experienced by Dr. DeParis. She wrote, "Looking back, I wonder if things may have been different if I'd sought professional help during residency, rather than 7 years later."

How we handle these difficult moments defines not only our personal journeys but also the collective strength of the medical community. By encouraging resilience and compassion, we can transform struggles into stepping stones toward healing and progress.

7.

Challenge the New Normal by Escaping Toxic Work Habits

Canceling self-care isn't heroic – it's harmful.

In a world where toxic work habits have become the norm, it's easy to mistake overcommitment for dedication. Checking emails at midnight, skipping dinner for deadlines, and working through lunch and weekends – these behaviors are often celebrated as markers of success. But the truth is simple: normalized toxicity is still toxic. Just because everyone does it doesn't mean it's normal or healthy. To truly thrive, we must redefine what it means to succeed at work.

At the heart of these toxic habits lies a disconnection – not just from balance or boundaries, but from ourselves. The incessant pull of "i" – iPhones, iPads, and other devices – has overshadowed the importance of reengaging with "I," our true selves. Disengaging from the distractions of our screens is perhaps the most important shift we can make. When we put down the devices and reconnect with our personal needs, values, and aspirations, we reclaim our time and rediscover fulfillment.

Start with the first hour of your day. If you're checking emails before your morning coffee, you're already surrendering your mental space to external demands. Instead, make the first hour sacred: journal, move, or simply breathe (I like to read and write). Establishing this boundary can set the tone for a healthier day. Similarly, the "working vacation" culture robs us of rest. Protect your time off by setting a vacation auto-reply and even deleting your email app for the duration.

Laptop lunches might seem efficient, but they kill focus and creativity. Taking real breaks in a new environment can do wonders for your productivity. And if you're trading bedtime stories with loved ones for emails, it's time to set a hard tech cutoff at 7 p.m. Being always reachable isn't sustainable either. Define what's urgent versus important and communicate your availability clearly to colleagues and clients.

A packed calendar without breaks is a recipe for burnout. Block off 15-20% of your day for deep, uninterrupted personal work. If the fear of being offline looms large, experiment with small steps – start with one-hour chunks of airplane mode. Stolen family moments can be reclaimed by creating tech-free zones at home. Teaching others to expect instant responses reinforces unhealthy habits; instead, wait 30 minutes before replying to most messages.

The inability to say no often stems from wanting to please everyone. Combat this by developing a decision framework for commitments. Likewise, not all notifications deserve your attention – turn off push notifications except for calls. Working Sundays to "get ahead" might seem productive, but scheduling joyful activities can bring balance to your weekends.

Feeling guilty about lunch breaks? Reframe them as essential by booking a daily walking meeting with yourself. Wearing "crazy busy" as a badge of honor perpetuates the problem. Replace vague busyness with clear priorities. Overwhelm is another silent killer – try a weekly audit to align your tasks with what truly matters.

False urgency is a common trap. Ask yourself, "What happens if this waits 24 hours?" The answer will often surprise you. Always-on culture can be addressed by setting boundaries in your email signature or specifying response times. Living in your inbox can consume your day; limit email checks to three times daily.

Breaking free from these habits, however, is easier said than done. Even with awareness and actionable suggestions, the ingrained nature of these behaviors often resists change. As the adage goes, old habits die hard. For many, the constant pull of technology resembles an addiction, making it all the more challenging to step away.

Understanding the addictive nature of internet and electronic use is key to addressing these behaviors. Notifications trigger dopamine responses in the brain, creating a reward loop that keeps us glued to our devices. Breaking this cycle requires deliberate effort and a structured approach. Rather than quitting cold turkey, which can be overwhelming, consider tapering your tech use with small, manageable changes.

Start by identifying the moments when your device use feels compulsive. Is it the first thing you reach for in the morning or a crutch during moments of boredom? Replace these triggers with healthier alternatives – like reading a book or practicing mindfulness. Gradually reduce the time spent on nonessential apps by setting app limits or scheduling device-free hours.

Creating boundaries can also help. Blurred work-life boundaries can be redefined with physical transition rituals, such as a walk to mark the end of your workday. If your home has become your office, create designated work-free spaces to protect your mental health, such as the dining table or bedroom. Honor these spaces as retreats from the digital world. Stack habits, like taking walking calls or squeezing in a quick workout during lunch. Turning off nonessential notifications and placing your phone in another room during focused tasks can also reduce the urge to check it constantly.

Accountability is another powerful tool. Share your goals with a friend or colleague and enlist their support in maintaining them. Celebrate small victories, like completing a workday without unnecessary screen time or enjoying a family dinner without interruptions.

The path to breaking free from toxic work habits and technology overuse may not be easy, but it is achievable. By taking incremental steps, we can reclaim our time, reconnect with our true selves, and create a healthier, more fulfilling relationship with both work and life.

8.

A Healthy Argument for – and Against – New and Expensive Drugs

Understanding the complex debate over drug costs.

The escalating costs of novel pharmaceuticals have sparked heated debates among stakeholders in health care, ranging from policymakers to clinicians and patients. Critics often focus on the prohibitively high price tags of these drugs, labeling them as burdensome to healthcare systems and individual patients. However, the conversation rarely accounts for the broader economic and clinical impacts of these therapies – specifically, their ability to offset other healthcare costs and deliver long-term value.

Understanding Cost Offsets in Medicine

Cost offsets refer to the savings generated in healthcare systems due to the use of certain interventions, which can reduce the need for other costly medical services. For example, a breakthrough drug for diabetes that effectively lowers HbA1c levels can prevent downstream complications such as diabetic nephropathy, cardiovascular disease, and amputations. By decreasing hospitalizations, surgeries, or long-term care, these drugs can offer significant economic advantages that justify their initial costs.

The hot button today is weight-loss drugs, like Ozempic. While most insurance plans cover Ozempic for diabetes management, coverage for FDA-unapproved use for weight loss is less common and varies widely depending on the plan. Without insurance, Ozempic can cost around $900 per month, making it a substantial expense for most individuals. However, studies suggest that significant weight loss achieved with Ozempic can lead to reduced healthcare costs associated with obesity-related complications like diabetes and cardiovascular issues.

In 2025, Independence Blue Cross, the Philadelphia, Pennsylvania region's largest health insurer, decided to no longer cover anti-obesity drugs like Ozempic when they're prescribed solely for weight loss. The drugs' high costs have caused an increase in premiums that "affect all members, whether they utilize weight loss drugs or not," the insurer said in a statement, and their policy is in line with other health insurers. Progressive talk show host Thom Hartmann retorted, "Americans are wondering out loud why we're getting ripped off by giant insurance companies when every other developed country in the world has healthcare as a right and pays an average of about half of what we do – and gets better outcomes."

Recently, the FDA approved tirzepatide (Zepbound) for adults with moderate-to-severe obstructive sleep apnea (OSA) and obesity (the improvement in OSA is likely related to body weight reduction). Used along with diet and exercise, this marks the first and only prescription medicine for OSA. Tirzepatide, which already holds indications for type 2 diabetes (Mounjaro) and chronic weight management, can be cost-prohibitive for many people. The list price without insurance or discounts is around $1000 per month. On the other hand, without treatment, OSA can lead to cardiovascular problems, mental health issues, car accidents from excessive daytime sleepiness, and many other consequences – all associated with very high long-term costs. Yet, health insurers are just as reluctant to cover Zepbound for OSA as they are Ozempic for obesity.

Data Supporting the Value of Expensive Medications

If we turn the temperature down and look to the research, numerous studies will demonstrate the cost-effectiveness of high-priced drugs in various medical domains. Take oncology, for instance. The advent of targeted therapies and immunotherapies, such as checkpoint inhibitors, has transformed the prognosis for several cancers. These drugs may significantly extend overall survival and progression-free survival compared to traditional chemotherapy. While the upfront costs are steep, the reduction in hospitalizations, emergency room visits, and palliative care expenses often compensates for the expenditure.

Breakthrough drugs – those representing an entirely new class of treatments – are especially worth the investment due to their transformative potential. Consider gene therapies like Zolgensma for spinal muscular atrophy in children under age 2. With a one-time-only single-dose price exceeding $2 million, it is one of the most expensive drugs ever developed. However, this therapy has been shown to dramatically improve survival and quality of life for affected children, potentially reducing or eliminating the need for lifelong supportive care, hospitalizations, and interventions. When viewed through the lens of cost offsets and quality-adjusted life years (QALYs), such drugs often represent a significant advancement in both healthcare outcomes and economic efficiency.

But there are also drugs of dubious value, not because they don't work, but because their price to value ratio is unconvincing, at least to policy decision-makers. For example, PCSK9 inhibitors, a class of drugs that lower levels of low-density lipoprotein (LDL) cholesterol, also known as "bad" cholesterol, have shown promise in reducing major cardiovascular events in patients with hypercholesterolemia who are statin-intolerant. However, a cost-effectiveness analysis published in *JAMA* highlighted that even considering their potential to avert myocardial infarctions, strokes, and associated healthcare costs over a patient's lifetime, this class of drugs as currently priced (>$14,000 per year) make them economically non-viable.

Critics argue that it is precisely the high cost of drugs that limits their accessibility, with insurers instituting barriers like prior authorization and "fail-first" policies that require patients to initially try and fail on cheaper drugs. While these measures aim to control costs, they often delay access to potentially life-saving therapies. My experience in both the insurance and pharmaceutical industries underscored the struggle between ensuring fiscal accountability and providing timely, equitable care.

Ethical Considerations and the Future of Innovation

The reality is that there are many types of drugs that show unequivocal safety and efficacy for a host of disorders in virtually all fields of medicine, but even with payer discounts of up to a third off retail price, they are not close to providing good value for money by conventional benchmarks. Medicine is then stuck with a choice between innovation, efficiency, and affordability, and this becomes an ethical dilemma rather than a therapeutic certainty.

The ethical dimension of pricing life-saving or life-altering drugs cannot be ignored. Ultimately, it means putting a price on how much a life is worth. The question of whether a drug is priced appropriately is difficult to determine. Still, pharmaceutical companies must ensure transparency in pricing strategies and prioritize patient access over profit margins. At the same time, society must recognize that innovation comes at a cost. Developing a new drug involves years of research, clinical trials, regulatory hurdles, and significant financial investment.

One solution is value-based pricing models, where the cost of a drug is tied to its real-world outcomes. Initiatives like these could help bridge the gap between pharmaceutical innovation and payer constraints, making high-value therapies more accessible. This approach may enable the discovery of future therapies that revolutionize care for diseases currently considered incurable.

A Balanced Perspective

The argument for new, expensive drugs lies not in defending the high prices themselves but in recognizing their broader value within the healthcare ecosystem. When such drugs are safe, effective, and groundbreaking, they often offset other costs, improve patient outcomes, and redefine standards of care. A balanced approach – embracing innovation while advocating for equitable access and sustainable pricing – will ensure that the promise of these therapies benefits all stakeholders. The true measure of a drug's worth extends beyond its price tag; it lies in its ability to save lives, alleviate suffering, and create a healthier future.

Yet, painful as it is to admit, physician researchers have observed that "draconian restrictions on access to drugs that are priced for profit maximization out of proportion to any value proposition and budget tolerances may continue to be the only way medicine can send a strong signal to innovators that their future rewards are tied not just to scientific advancement but also to affordability. This is not just an issue for pharmaceutical companies. Profit maximation behavior in medicine out of proportion to value provided is widespread. Ultimately, this message will need to be heeded by the entire health care enterprise."

9.

Flights of Fancy

How doctors soar – or stay grounded
– informs their ability to heal and connect.

The ability to fly is one of the most studied developments in science and engineering. Richard Dawkins' 2021 book, *Flights of Fancy*, is perhaps the definitive work on the subject. From the deadly dance between moths and bats, to the wonders of airplanes, this book examines nature's desire to break free from the bonds of gravity (or, as Dawkins says in the closing lines of the book, nature's escape from gravity into the third dimension). These moments, though sometimes brief and ungainly, have nevertheless provided safety, threat and wonder in equal measure to those who have learned flight's secrets.

Although Dawkins extensively covers both natural and mechanized flight, he omits the most interesting type of flight, in my estimation: flights of fancy of the human mind. By this I mean, for example, the "Walter Mitty" syndrome. Walter Mitty syndrome is a term used to describe someone who indulges in fantastic daydreams of personal triumphs. The term comes from the character Walter Mitty in James Thurber's short story, "The Secret Life of Walter Mitty," which was first published in *The New Yorker* in 1939.

James Thurber's Mitty is a nebbish who is conscripted into mundane tasks, such as chauffeuring his demanding wife on errands, including weekend shopping excursions. He escapes his humdrum existence through his imagination, pretending to be various daring and heroic characters, such as a bomber pilot, Navy commander, and surgeon, among others.

A surgeon?

I must have it backwards. I thought doctors were the real daydreamers, reflecting their desire for excitement and escape, contrasting with what over time becomes a rather ordinary life.

Indeed, doctors might seem an unlikely group to exhibit "Walter Mitty" tendencies. After all, the medical profession carries an inherent drama – life-and-death decisions, profound human connections, and the constant march of discovery. Yet, the very intensity of this world often prompts physicians to indulge in their own flights of fancy. These imaginative escapes might involve envisioning a perfect clinical outcome, dreaming of professional acclaim, or even longing for lives entirely separate from medicine's relentless demands.

The paradox of the physician daydreamer is rooted in the gap between expectation and reality. For many doctors, the journey begins with idealistic aspirations of healing, adventure, and intellectual mastery. However, as years of training transform into decades of practice, the reality sets in: endless paperwork, administrative burdens, and routine cases outnumber the heroic saves or cutting-edge breakthroughs. Even the thrilling moments often come packaged in exhaustion and the weight of responsibility. Thus, the mind begins to wander, conjuring alternative worlds that offer the excitement, validation, or simplicity that reality cannot.

This tendency isn't a weakness; it's a survival mechanism. Daydreams can serve as a counterbalance to medicine's grueling demands, a necessary recalibration that allows the practitioner to remain connected to their humanity. A surgeon imagining themselves as a daring explorer or a pioneering inventor isn't so different from a child pretending to be a superhero. These mental excursions rekindle creativity, buoy spirits, and provide a safe space for aspirations that might otherwise wither under the daily grind and routine of practicing medicine.

There is, however, a pathological version of the Walter Mitty syndrome. The term may also refer to maladaptive daydreaming, a disorder characterized by excessive daydreaming that can be damaging to one's well-being. Symptoms of maladaptive daydreaming include vivid daydreams, long daydreaming sessions, daydreams triggered by real-life events, daydreaming sessions that interrupt sleep, and repetitive motions or whisperings while daydreaming.

This irrational side of the Walter Mitty syndrome takes the idea of flights of fancy to an extreme where they cease to be mere escapes and become barriers to functional living. Maladaptive daydreaming, first described by psychologist Eli Somer in 2002, can dominate an individual's mental landscape, consuming hours of their day and interfering with personal, academic, or professional responsibilities. Unlike the brief, whimsical escapes most people enjoy, maladaptive daydreamers are caught in a loop of vivid, immersive fantasies that can feel more fulfilling or compelling than reality itself.

The triggers for these daydreams are often tied to emotional needs – loneliness, stress, or dissatisfaction. Real-life events, music, or visual cues can act as catalysts, pulling individuals into elaborate inner worlds. While these daydreams may provide temporary relief or a sense of control, the cost is significant: missed opportunities, fractured relationships, and, in severe cases, an inability to distinguish between fantasy and reality.

For physicians, who are often under immense pressure, there's a cautionary tale here. The same imaginative flights that can provide solace or inspiration might, if unchecked, turn into distractions or coping mechanisms that hinder their ability to engage fully with patients or their own lives. For instance, the doctor who constantly fantasizes about a different career might struggle to find meaning in their current one, leaving them disillusioned or burned out. Similarly, the mental exhaustion of caregiving might push a practitioner toward unhealthy escapism, making it harder to connect with the real challenges and triumphs of their work.

Recognizing the line between healthy and maladaptive daydreaming is crucial – not just for individuals but for the systems and communities around them. Physicians, like others, need support structures that allow for healthy expression and acknowledgment of stressors without pushing them toward isolation or unproductive coping mechanisms. Encouraging reflective practices, engaging with mentors, and providing space for creative outlets can help channel the flights of fancy in constructive ways, ensuring they inspire rather than impede.

Ultimately, the difference between a healthy Walter Mitty moment and maladaptive daydreaming lies in its impact. When flights of fancy lift us briefly, they serve as a reminder of human creativity and resilience. When they ground us in dissatisfaction or disconnection, they demand attention and intervention. Like all forms of flight, whether physical or metaphorical, the aim is not merely to soar but to land safely and with purpose.

10.

What if Transitions of Care Resembled Transitions of Power?

Examining presidential transitions can provide valuable insights into how we might improve the continuity and quality of care for patients.

The peaceful transition of power to the 47th president of the U.S. occurred January 6, 2025. It was the loser of the presidential election who ironically ensured an orderly process and certified the results.

In medicine, transitions of care – whether from inpatient to skilled nursing facility, from hospital to home, or during the passing of responsibility from one practitioner to another – represent pivotal moments in the continuity of patient treatment. These handoffs, rife with potential for miscommunication and error, are reminiscent of historical transitions of power in the U.S., where the stakes are equally high and the outcomes often uncertain.

By drawing parallels between these two domains, we can illuminate both the pitfalls and the promise inherent in such critical junctures.

The Assassination Scenario: Chaos and Urgency

When a president is assassinated, as with Abraham Lincoln or John F. Kennedy, the transfer of power is abrupt and fraught with chaos. Similarly, a sudden transition of care can occur when a physician becomes unexpectedly unavailable, such as in an emergency or abrupt resignation. The handoff of patient care responsibilities between medical students, residents, or attending physicians during shift changes can also resemble the abrupt and often chaotic transitions of power following an unexpected event, such as the assassination of a president.

In these moments, the incoming provider – like Andrew Johnson or Lyndon B. Johnson – must quickly establish authority, absorb the context of the situation, and steer the ship without prior preparation. Just as Lyndon Johnson had to navigate the minefields of the Civil Rights Movement and Vietnam War immediately upon taking office, an incoming physician must rapidly assimilate critical patient details while simultaneously making urgent medical decisions. The potential for mistakes is immense, but so too is the opportunity for decisive leadership.

The Resignation: Precipitous Departures

The resignation of Richard Nixon in 1974 brought Gerald Ford to power under unusual and destabilizing circumstances. In medicine, this could be likened to a physician stepping away due to illness or other personal reasons, leaving behind unresolved patient issues. Gerald Ford's task of restoring public trust parallels the challenge faced by a covering physician who must address both the unfinished tasks and the skepticism of patients and colleagues alike. Ford's handling of the aftermath serves as a reminder that even in suboptimal conditions, stability can be restored with clear communication and steady leadership.

The Lame Duck: Minimal Engagement

A president nearing the end of their term – a "lame duck" – may become less engaged with the day-to-day responsibilities of governance. This can be mirrored in a physician going on vacation, nearing retirement, or transitioning to a new role, whose diminished investment might affect the quality of patient care.

For example, a hospitalist or locum tenens physicians who knows they are leaving at the end of the month might intentionally delay addressing complex issues, leaving a larger burden for their successor. Just as the transition from Herbert Hoover to Franklin D. Roosevelt during the Great Depression highlighted the risks of disengagement, so too can a lackadaisical handoff in medicine exacerbate challenges for incoming providers.

The Refusal to Transition: Contested Handovers

Donald Trump's refusal to concede the 2020 election epitomizes the dangers of a contested transition of power. In health care, this could be paralleled by providers who resist relinquishing control, either out of pride, mistrust, or a sense of unfinished business.

For instance, an outgoing physician may be reluctant to transfer a long-term patient to another provider, withholding crucial details or undermining the new caregiver's authority. The resultant friction can compromise patient outcomes, much as contested political transitions strain national stability.

The Harmonious Transfer: Similar Paradigms

When power transitions from one political party to another – as from Jimmy Carter to Ronald Reagan, George H.W. Bush to Bill Clinton, or Barack Obama to Donald Trump – it often signals a dramatic shift in priorities and policies. In medicine, this can resemble a patient's care transitioning between practitioners with differing philosophies.

For example, a holistic, patient-centered physician may transfer care to a more data-driven clinician, or vice versa. Such ideological contrasts can disorient patients and caregivers alike, requiring deliberate efforts to reconcile divergent approaches to ensure continuity of care.

However, transitions can be harmonious despite political differences. Consider the transfer of power from President Dwight D. Eisenhower (Republican) to John F. Kennedy (Democrat). Both parties worked to ensure a seamless handover for the good of the nation.

Similarly, in health care, detailed discharge planning, comprehensive medication reconciliation, and effective communication between hospital staff and receiving facilities are essential to prevent errors and ensure patients continue to receive the appropriate level of care.

The goal is to maintain stability and continuity, minimizing the risk of complications or readmissions, analogous to maintaining constancy during a change in leadership.

Leadership and Politics in Health Care

The critical role of leadership and politics in health care cannot be overstated. Just as political transitions depend on the vision, competence, and stability of incoming leaders, the success of transitions in care relies heavily on strong leadership within medical teams and institutions. Leaders in health care set the tone for collaboration, advocate for resources, and implement systems that minimize errors during transitions.

Moreover, health care politics – from hospital administration to national health policy – play a pivotal role in shaping how care transitions are managed. Policies that prioritize patient safety, incentivize effective communication, and provide adequate staffing are as essential to health care as bipartisan cooperation is to governance. In both realms, leadership determines whether transitions lead to progress or regression, continuity or disruption.

Lessons from History

Historical transitions of power offer critical lessons for improving transitions of care. Just as the United States has developed protocols for the peaceful transfer of power – such as the swearing-in of vice presidents, the sharing of intelligence briefings, and the preparation of transition teams – health care can benefit from standardized procedures and collaborative practices. These might include detailed discharge summaries, structured sign-out protocols (e.g., SBAR: Situation, Background, Assessment, Recommendation), and robust communication channels.

Moreover, empathy and foresight are as vital in medicine as they are in governance. Leaders who recognize the gravity of transitions – and approach them with humility and preparation – can lessen risks and pave the way for success. Whether in the Oval Office or the operating room, the true measure of a transition lies not in the smoothness of the process but in its capacity to safeguard those most affected.

A Shared Responsibility

Ultimately, transitions – whether of care or power – are a shared responsibility. They demand not only the competence of the incoming leader or practitioner but also the cooperation and goodwill of the outgoing party. By acknowledging the parallels between these spheres, we can better appreciate the duties of both and strive to handle them with the grace they deserve. In doing so, we honor the trust placed in us – by citizens or patients – to guide them safely through uncertainty to stability and hope.

11.

It Was a Very Good Year – Or Was It?

The ingredients of a very good year vary but often center on health and wellness.

Frank Sinatra's 1965 hit, "It Was a Very Good Year," framed the benchmarks of a life well-lived through relationships at various ages: when he was 17, "small-town girls ... on the village green"; at 21, "city girls who lived up the stair"; at 35, "blue-blooded girls of independent means."

Fast forward 60 years. What are the ingredients that now constitute "a very good year?" Data from a survey of 2,000 Americans offers an intriguing snapshot: the average rating for 2024 was a 6.1 out of 10, a score that captures a sense of cautious optimism amid the mundane.

An Average Year with Bright Spots

The most common score given was a neutral five out of 10, indicating a year that was neither particularly bad nor exceptionally good. Yet, 30% of respondents rated their year as an eight or higher, suggesting significant pockets of positivity. At the heart of many memorable moments in 2024 were connections, growth, and personal achievements.

When asked what made the year stand out, the most popular response was deeply heartwarming: reconnecting with an old friend or family member. This simple yet meaningful act underscores the enduring value of relationships in defining life's quality. Other notable experiences included creative and personal growth, getting a new pet, learning a new skill, volunteering for a cause, and addressing health and wellness goals. Collectively, these responses reflect a shift toward valuing personal enrichment and relational depth over purely material accomplishments.

Themes of Personal Growth

Growth was a recurring theme. An impressive 67% of respondents felt they experienced growth in some form during the year, with over half citing improvements in their personal lives. Of those who say they did do some growing in 2024, over half (52%) felt they'd seen improvements in their personal life, while 38% saw developments in their mental and emotional life and 29% felt they'd made improvements in their physical health and fitness. Financial strides were also noted, with 25% reporting improvements in their monetary situations.

This emphasis on growth aligns with a broader cultural trend: the pursuit of self-improvement as a marker of a fulfilling life. Learning new skills, dealing with health challenges, and paying off significant debts were among the milestones celebrated, demonstrating resilience and a focus on long-term goals.

Memorable Moments Beyond Growth

Other standout events included visiting new places, starting new jobs, and even purchasing significant items like a car. These experiences highlight the importance of novelty and milestones in creating a sense of accomplishment. Once-in-a-lifetime events, such as witnessing an eclipse or attending a memorable concert, also featured prominently, emphasizing the human desire for unique and enriching experiences.

The Numbers Behind the Year

The detailed breakdown of scores paints a refined picture:

- **Scores of 1-4:** About 23% of respondents rated their year below average, indicating struggles or unmet expectations.
- **Scores of 5-7:** The majority, 47%, landed in the middle range, suggesting a year that balanced challenges with positive moments.
- **Scores of 8-10:** A notable 30% rated their year as excellent, reflecting significant personal or professional successes.

Reflections on a "Good" Year

What makes a year "very good" in the modern era? Unlike Sinatra's romantic benchmarks, today's metrics lean heavily on connection, growth, resilience, and health. From tackling mental health challenges to achieving fitness and wellness goals, health remains a cornerstone of a fulfilling year: of the top 20 events that made 2024 "memorable," overcoming a significant health challenge ranked 7. Achieving a fitness goal and quitting smoking ranked 11 and 18, respectively. Reuniting with loved ones and accomplishing personal goals factored significantly in defining a fulfilling year. As uncertainty reigns in the world, these themes offer a roadmap for finding meaning and satisfaction, regardless of external circumstances.

Politics was surprising absent among the responses despite dominating much of the headlines for the year. In 2024, the benchmark for "a very good year" seemed to lie not in perfection or political penchant, but in progress – in small, meaningful moments that remind us of our capacity to adapt, grow, and connect. Perhaps, like Sinatra crooning about his years of wine and roses, we too can find the poetry in our decidedly modern lives and look forward to a future consisting of vintage years.

12.

Moving Beyond the Binary to Redefine Well-Being

Dopamine is linked to well-being,
and well-being is linked to inclusive mental health care.

Dopamine is a vital neurotransmitter that plays a crucial role in the brain's reward system, influencing pleasure, motivation, and movement. Often referred to as the "feel-good" chemical, dopamine is released during enjoyable activities, reinforcing behaviors that lead to rewards and driving individuals to pursue goals. It is essential for coordinating smooth movements; a deficiency in dopamine causes Parkinson's disease.

Additionally, dopamine contributes to cognitive functions such as learning and memory, impacting attention and focus. Imbalances in dopamine levels can lead to various mental health issues, including depression, schizophrenia, and addiction, highlighting its significance in overall well-being.

Choose Your Dopamine

Fake Dopamine	Real Dopamine
Binge-watch TV	Catch sunrise
Mindless scrolling	Prayer/Meditation
Junk food	Sip healthy tea
Overdrink coffee	Walk with friends
Work without rest	Exercise/Yoga
Unneeded shopping	Read
Over-yesing	Slow down
Gossiping	Rest
All-night gaming	Deep breathing
Late-night phone use	Cooking healthy meals
Procrastinating	Music/Art/Creativity

The "Choose Your Dopamine" chart (above) appears in many basic psychological textbooks. It attempts to guide individuals toward healthier habits by categorizing activities into "Fake" and "Real" sources of dopamine. However, its simplistic and dichotomous framework raises critical concerns. Such categorizations risk shaming individuals for their choices, ignoring the diversity of lived experiences and the nuances of mental health.

For example, labeling activities like binge-watching TV or late-night gaming as "fake" dopamine disregards the genuine joy, comfort, and community many derive from these activities. Neurodivergent individuals, in particular, often find meaning and connection through interests like fandoms, which foster creativity, self-expression, and friendships. Online gaming, another activity dismissed as unhealthy in the chart, serves as a critical social outlet for many, helping build lasting friendships and even romantic relationships.

By promoting a narrow standard for "healthy" habits, this chart perpetuates a one-size-fits-all approach to mental health, which fails to account for individual differences. It also overlooks the broader systemic challenges – ableism, racism, classism, and other forms of oppression – that significantly impact mental health. Too often, these societal barriers are ignored in favor of blaming individuals for their struggles, further marginalizing those who cannot adhere to traditional definitions of well-being.

Ultimately, the most "real" dopamine comes from exercising autonomy in one's choices, free from judgment or imposed standards. Mental health care must move beyond oversimplified frameworks and focus on creating inclusive, compassionate approaches that respect individual needs and circumstances.

Moving beyond oversimplified frameworks like the one presented in the "Choose Your Dopamine" chart begins with recognizing that mental health is deeply intertwined with social and cultural factors. A person's habits and coping mechanisms cannot be evaluated in isolation from the context in which they live. For example, individuals facing oppression or economic hardship may rely on activities like gaming or binge-watching TV as accessible and affordable ways to find joy or connection. Mental health professionals must acknowledge and validate these coping mechanisms rather than dismissing them as "fake."

Inclusive mental health care also requires a shift away from judgmental narratives that prescribe universal standards of well-being. Instead, mental health providers should adopt a person-centered approach, focusing on the unique needs, preferences, and goals of each individual. This means asking patients what brings them joy, connection, and meaning, rather than imposing preconceived notions of what is "healthy." For some, this might involve traditional practices like meditation or exercise; for others, it might include creative activities, virtual communities, or hobbies that are often stigmatized. The emphasis should be on whether these activities enhance the individual's overall sense of well-being and connectedness.

Compassionate mental health care must also address the structural barriers that contribute to mental health challenges. It is not enough to encourage self-care practices without acknowledging the impact of systemic inequities such as those mentioned above. Mental health professionals and advocates should work to dismantle these barriers by promoting policies and practices that increase access to care, reduce stigma, and create more equitable environments. This includes ensuring that mental health resources are affordable, culturally sensitive, and accessible to marginalized communities.

Education and training for mental health providers should also prioritize cultural humility and an understanding of neurodiversity. Providers must be equipped to work with individuals whose experiences and coping strategies may differ from their own. This includes valuing and supporting the unique ways neurodivergent individuals perceive the world and acknowledging the strengths they bring to their communities. By celebrating diversity and moving away from rigid definitions of "normal" or "abnormal," mental health care can better serve all individuals.

Finally, mental health care must move toward a strengths-based model that empowers individuals rather than pathologizing their choices. This means focusing on what works for each person and helping them build on their existing sources of resilience and fulfillment. By creating safe spaces where individuals feel seen, heard, and respected, mental health providers can instill a deeper sense of trust and collaboration. In turn, this allows individuals to explore new ways of enhancing their well-being without fear of judgment or shame. Everyone's journey toward well-being is different, and by respecting individual needs and circumstances, the field can better support people in finding their own paths to healing and fulfillment.

13.

Workplace Relationships: Colleagues, Confidants, or More?

Navigating relationships in medical settings can be a tricky "affair."

The medical workplace is a unique environment. Long hours, high drama, and shared challenges create opportunities for connection, collaboration, and occasionally, conflict. As physicians and other medical professionals develop these relationships, they often find themselves grappling with questions: Are colleagues simply allies in a shared professional mission? Can they also be confidants and close friends? And what happens when romantic relationships develop in this high-pressure, hierarchical setting? Exploring these dynamics reveals a spectrum of possibilities, each with implications for individuals and treatment teams.

Friendships in the Workplace: Strengths and Challenges

For most professionals, workplace relationships are primarily about shared goals and mutual respect. Medicine, with its emphasis on teamwork, highlights this dynamic even more. Physicians often rely on one another to deliver patient care effectively, making collaboration essential. These relationships are inherently professional, dictated by the job rather than personal choice.

Maintaining healthy boundaries is a cornerstone of effective workplace interactions. Overly personal connections can blur the lines between professional responsibilities and personal relationships, potentially complicating team dynamics. In larger teams or hierarchical environments, where differences in roles and authority are pronounced, such entanglements can lead to misunderstandings or even ethical concerns.

However, some argue that the hours spent together – often under intense conditions – inevitably foster deeper connections. Shared experiences and common struggles can create bonds that transcend professional boundaries, offering emotional support and camaraderie. In these cases, workplace friendships may enhance morale, build trust, and improve overall team performance. Yet even in these positive scenarios, maintaining professionalism is critical to preserving respect and balance.

Romantic Relationships: A Double-Edged Sword

The intense environment of medical practice can also give rise to romantic relationships. When balanced and consensual, these connections can provide much-needed emotional support, grounding professionals amid the stresses of their demanding careers. In some cases, such relationships may even strengthen collaboration, as shared goals and mutual understanding drive both partners forward.

Yet, romantic relationships in the workplace, particularly in medicine, are fraught with challenges. Power imbalances – such as those between faculty and residents or attendings and medical students – are a significant concern. Even when both parties enter the relationship willingly, differences in authority and career stage can create ethical dilemmas and leave one party vulnerable. The perception of favoritism or coercion can erode team trust and lead to workplace conflicts.

Age gaps and differing life stages often exacerbate these challenges. Colleagues may question the appropriateness of such relationships, and the individuals involved may struggle with mismatched expectations or priorities. Institutions typically implement policies to manage these dynamics, but even with guidelines in place, the emotional and ethical complexities remain.

Medical Marriages

About 85% of physicians are married, and nearly 20% are married to other doctors. Medical marriages illustrate perhaps the deepest connection of personal and professional lives in the field of healthcare. While the demands can be immense, such relationships also offer the promise of intense understanding and support – an anchor in the often turbulent waters of medical practice. For these couples – many who meet as medical students – the key to thriving lies in rewarding time and a shared commitment to a life in medicine together.

However, medical marriages also pose challenges. The alignment of demanding careers can strain relationships, particularly when partners work long hours, cover night shifts, or are on call. Burnout, a prevalent issue in healthcare, may impact both individuals simultaneously, leaving little room for one partner to support the other. The intensity of the profession may also lead to competition, especially when both partners are striving for leadership roles, prestigious positions, or recognition in their fields.

Research has shown time and again that keys to success and resilience in medical marriages are open communication, compromise (hint: joint decision-making), and meticulous planning. Without these three factors, spouses of physicians run the risk of being made to feel less than or second to a career in medicine.

Setting Boundaries: The Foundation of Professional Relationships

Whether navigating friendships, alliances, or romantic relationships, setting boundaries is essential. Boundaries protect personal and professional integrity, ensuring that interactions remain respectful and productive. In the case of workplace friendships, this means balancing connection with professionalism – sharing enough to foster trust without overstepping into personal territory.

For romantic relationships, boundaries involve understanding and adhering to institutional policies, disclosing relationships when necessary, and maintaining professionalism during work hours. Transparency, mutual respect, and a commitment to ethical conduct can help mitigate the risks of workplace romances.

Workplace Culture: The Invisible Hand

The culture of a workplace plays a pivotal role in shaping relationships. In small, tight-knit teams, close connections may naturally develop, enhancing collaboration and creating a supportive environment. Conversely, in larger or more competitive settings, professionals may feel the need to maintain greater distance, focusing more on individual achievements than team cohesion.

Leaders have a critical responsibility to model healthy boundaries and foster a culture of respect. By encouraging open communication and providing guidance on managing workplace relationships, they can create an environment where individuals feel valued and supported without compromising professionalism.

The Bigger Picture: Balancing Connection and Professionalism

Workplace relationships, whether professional, friendly, or romantic, are integral to the medical field. They shape how teams function, how care is delivered, and how individuals experience their careers. While friendships and romances can enrich the workplace, they require careful navigation to avoid pitfalls.

For physicians, whose roles demand both empathy and professionalism, the risks and rewards are particularly high. The key lies in forming relationships that prioritize respect, maintain boundaries, and support both personal and professional growth. By striking this balance, medical professionals can create a workplace where individuals and teams can thrive – proving that colleagues can indeed be allies, confidants, or more, provided the relationship serves both integrity and purpose.

Section 2:

The Multiverse

14.

A Brief Overview of AI in Medicine

The intersection of AI and medical practice promises to revolutionize patient care and redefine the boundaries of medicine.

The 1956 Dartmouth Artificial Intelligence conference is often credited as the seminal event that gave birth to the field of AI. Organized by mathematician John McCarthy, this gathering brought together some of the leading minds of the time to explore a variety of advanced research topics. These included complexity theory, language simulation, neuron nets, abstraction of content from sensory inputs, the relationship of randomness to creative thinking, and learning machines.

McCarthy coined the term "Artificial Intelligence" to describe this novel area of study, which promised to harness information technology for the benefit of humanity. The conference marked the beginning of a journey that would continually shape the development of AI and influence generations of scientists.

There is no specific record of medical doctors being part of this initial conference, as the intersection of AI and medicine became more prominent in later years as the technology developed. What follows is an exploration of important timelines, key figures, landmark projects, controversies, achievements, and potential future directions in this dynamic intersection.

Early Beginnings and Initial Developments

The intersection of artificial intelligence and medicine began to take shape in the 1970s, with the development of expert systems designed to assist in clinical decision-making. One of the earliest and most notable projects was MYCIN, a knowledge-based computer consultation program developed in 1972 at Stanford University by Edward H. (Ted) Shortliffe,

MD, PhD, which aimed to diagnose bacterial infections and recommend antibiotics. Although MYCIN was never implemented in clinical practice due to various limitations, it demonstrated the potential of AI in medicine and inspired further research. Studies showed that MYCIN's advice was comparable to that of infectious disease experts.

Advancements in the 1980s and 1990s

Throughout the 1980s and 1990s, AI in medicine expanded with systems like INTERNIST-I and its successor, Quick Medical Reference (QMR), which focused on diagnosing complex internal medicine cases. These systems highlighted the challenges of integrating AI in clinical environments, including issues related to data quality, system complexity, and clinician acceptance. Despite these hurdles, the period was marked by significant advancements in computational power and algorithm development, setting the stage for more sophisticated applications.

Expansion of AI in Imaging and Diagnostics

The 1990s saw the application of AI in medical imaging, with algorithms being developed to interpret X-rays, CT scans, and MRIs. The advent of machine learning techniques further enhanced the accuracy of diagnostic tools. Systems like CADx (Computer-Aided Diagnosis) began assisting radiologists in identifying conditions such as cancer, significantly improving early detection rates. Over time, CADx systems have evolved to become more complex, capable of detecting subtle abnormalities that may be difficult for the human eye to see.

The Rise of Machine Learning and Data-Driven Approaches

The late 1990s and early 2000s saw a greater shift towards machine learning and data-driven approaches, fueled by the increasing availability of digital health records and biomedical data. Projects like IBM's Watson, which gained fame for winning "Jeopardy!" in 2011, were adapted for healthcare applications, such as cancer treatment recommendations. These efforts demonstrated AI's potential to analyze vast datasets and support personalized medicine, though they also faced scrutiny regarding accuracy and transparency.

The AI Renaissance: Deep Learning and Personalized Medicine

The 2010s marked a turning point with the advent of deep learning. Algorithms like Convolutional Neural Networks (CNNs) revolutionized image recognition, leading to breakthroughs in pathology and radiology. AI tools began to predict patient outcomes, personalize treatments, and optimize clinical workflows. One notable project included Google DeepMind's application of AI in ophthalmology to detect many forms of macular disease affecting the retina.

Controversies and Challenges

Despite remarkable achievements, AI's integration into medicine has been fraught with controversy. Criticisms include biases in training datasets, lack of transparency in algorithmic decision-making, concerns over data privacy, and the potential for AI to exacerbate healthcare inequalities. For example, an algorithm containing a "race factor" lead to an overestimation of kidney function in Black patients, potentially delaying diagnosis and treatment of their kidney disease by making it appear less severe than it actually was. In some instances, patients died waiting for kidney transplants because they were not given sufficient priority on waiting lists.

The deployment of IBM Watson for oncology faced scrutiny over inaccuracies and its limited clinical utility. Indeed, a review of 519 studies of AI in health care revealed major shortcomings in the consideration of real patient care data in applications. These incidents underscored the need for rigorous validation and ethical oversight in developing AI-driven healthcare solutions. The transparency of AI decision-making processes and the ethical implications of relying on machine-based recommendations are ongoing debates within non-medical fields as well.

Current Accomplishments

Criticisms notwithstanding, AIs impact on medicine today is undeniable. It is transforming areas such as drug discovery, telemedicine, and predictive analytics. Tools like AI-powered chatbots enhance patient engagement, while algorithms predict disease outbreaks and optimize public health strategies. Moreover, robotic surgery systems like Da Vinci Surgical System leverage AI to improve precision and outcomes in the operating room. The da Vinci system is used for a variety of procedures, including prostatectomies, cardiac valve repair, and renal and gynecologic surgeries.

Future Directions

Looking ahead, the future of AI in medicine is promising, with potential breakthroughs in genomics, drug discovery, and personalized treatment. The integration of AI with other technologies, such as the Internet of Things (IoT) and blockchain, could further transform healthcare delivery. The use of blockchain technology enhances the security and privacy of the data produced by IoT healthcare devices. It guarantees the privacy of sensitive health information while granting authorized parties access to relevant information when needed.

As AI continues to evolve, it will likely play an increasingly integral role in shaping the future of medicine. Key areas of focus include:

- **Explainable AI (XAI):** Developing transparent algorithms to foster trust among healthcare providers and patients.
- **Integration with Genomics:** Leveraging AI to unlock insights from genetic data, advancing personalized medicine.
- **AI in Mental Health:** Using natural language processing and sentiment analysis to enhance diagnosis and treatment of mental health conditions.
- **Ethical AI Development:** Establishing robust frameworks to address biases, ensure equitable access, and safeguard patient data.

Balancing Innovation and Oversight

Legal constraints will undoubtedly shape the future of AI, particularly in sensitive areas like medicine. The evolving regulatory landscape reflects growing concerns about safety, fairness, accountability, and the ethical use of AI technologies.

Effective regulation must strike a balance between fostering innovation and protecting public interests. Policymakers face the dual challenge of preventing harm while ensuring AI's transformative potential is not stifled. A cooperative approach involving both state and federal actors, alongside industry and academic input, is essential to navigate the complexities of AI governance. While state-level laws will focus on issues of specific interest to individual states, the trend points toward federal leadership in creating comprehensive AI regulations where national standards are crucial for consistency and public trust.

Conclusion

AI in medicine has untapped potential, but it must be tempered by the challenges of ethical implementation. As technology continues to evolve, its ability to improve patient care, reduce costs, and enhance outcomes will depend on collaboration between AI experts, healthcare providers, and policymakers. This partnership will ensure that AI serves as a powerful ally in advancing the future of medicine, and in many ways, it mirrors the multidisciplinary undertaking at Dartmouth nearly 70 years ago – only now with doctors included.

15.

AI for *Time's* Person of the Year

The transformative potential of AI in medicine parallels visionary themes in science fiction, going where no one has gone before – not even Time magazine.

2024 was a missed opportunity for *Time* magazine. The short list for *Time's* 2024 Person of the Year was mostly a distressing list of podcasters, politicians, and other peddlers: Joe Rogan, Elon Musk, Mark Zuckerberg, and of course the obligatory 2024 presidential pretenders Kamala Harris and Donald Trump (Trump, the winner, was also *Time's* Person of the Year in 2016).

Time began announcing its person of the year – actually, "man" of the year – in 1927 to acknowledge "the individual who most shaped the headlines over the previous 12 months, for better or for worse." *Time's* editor-in-chief Sam Jacobs provided insight into the selections over the years.

"As a tradition, Person of the Year springs from the Great Man Theory of history, a belief that individuals have the power to transform society," Jacobs wrote. "The selections over the years have tended to follow certain patterns. The person chosen has typically been a ruler over traditional domains of power."

Time has considered primarily world leaders, dignitaries, and cultural figures – and an occasional celebrity. The 2023 Person of the Year was a popstar. Quick, can you name the person?

Too late. It was Taylor Swift. It just goes to show how insignificant *Time's* picks can be despite Swift's successful Eras tour of 2023-2024.

I suppose the editors at *Time* knew their choices might quickly fade from public consciousness, so they decided to expanded the category around the turn of the century to include an idea, concept, object, or group

– for example, Whistleblowers (2002), Protestors (2011), Silence Breakers (#MeToo in 2017), and Guardians (2018).

With this expansion in mind, I would have cast my vote in 2024 for AI – a concept, but really a conglomerate of all categories, except "people," of course.

AI was the most talked about and hyped development of 2024, transforming operations across numerous sectors, from manufacturing to financial services. AI ushered in groundbreaking advancements in several areas of medicine, assisting doctors, and in my specialty of psychiatry, posing as therapists.

AI systems that possess the ability to understand, learn, and apply knowledge across a wide range of tasks at a level comparable to human intelligence – so-called Artificial General Intelligence (AGI) – are the ones to keep an eye on. Unlike narrow AI, which is designed for specific tasks, AGI is capable of performing any intellectual task that a human can. The development of AGI is a major goal in the field of AI research, but it remains largely theoretical at this point, as current AI systems are specialized and lack the generalization capabilities of human cognition.

AGI is not a new idea. I was watching an episode of the original Star Trek series – "What Are Little Girls Made Of" – which first aired in 1966. The promise of AGI was featured, although it was not called that by name. Dr. Roger Korby, a brilliant yet morally compromised scientist, attempts to achieve human immortality by transferring consciousness into android bodies, ultimately surpassing the limits of humanity and identity. Such a feat involves multiple disciplines, including computer science, neuroscience, philosophy, and ethics. Surely AGI should garner accolades and long overdue recognition as *Time's* Person of the Year.

AGI is an especially compelling force in medicine due to its potential to revolutionize healthcare delivery, diagnostics, and patient care. In theory, AGI could analyze vast amounts of medical data far more quickly and accurately than human practitioners, leading to more precise diagnoses and personalized treatment plans. This capability could enhance decision-making in complex cases by integrating information from diverse sources, including genetic data, medical history, and real-time patient monitoring.

Furthermore, AGI could significantly improve the efficiency of clinical workflows by automating routine tasks, allowing healthcare professionals to focus more on direct patient care. It could also facilitate the development of new medical technologies and therapies by identifying patterns and insights that are challenging for humans to discern.

If you are convinced there is a place for AGI in the future, I suggest you watch an episode of Star Trek with a contrasting view: "The Ultimate Computer." An advanced artificially intelligent control system, the M-5 Multitronic unit, is capable of operating the Enterprise with only a skeleton crew. However, M-5 malfunctions and engages in real war rather than simulated war. Captain Kirk disables M-5, but he must gamble on the humanity of an opposing starship captain to not retaliate against the Enterprise.

Kirk tells Mr. Spock that he knew the other captain personally and was certain he would show compassion and not fire upon them. Dr. McCoy adds: "Compassion. That's the one thing no machine ever had."

Perhaps AI does need more persona before we can consider it for *Time's* Person of the Year.

16.

Can AI Help Me Become a Better Version of Myself?

The journey of self-improvement in medicine never ends.

Doctors hold a unique place in society, entrusted with the well-being of their patients, and this privilege comes with the constant challenge of striving to be better versions of themselves. The journey toward personal and professional growth for physicians begins with self-awareness. Recognizing one's strengths and areas for improvement is critical, as medicine is as much an art as it is a science. Reflection on clinical encounters, soliciting feedback from colleagues, and engaging in practices like journaling or narrative medicine can help doctors better understand their patterns, biases, and emotional responses. This process of introspection lays the foundation for meaningful change.

Recognizing and Addressing Bias

Doctors must recognize and address several biases to provide equitable and effective care. Implicit bias, rooted in unconscious stereotypes about race, gender, age, or socioeconomic status, can lead to disparities in diagnosis, treatment, and outcomes. Confirmation bias, the tendency to favor information that aligns with pre-existing beliefs, can hinder accurate clinical decision-making. Anchoring bias, or relying too heavily on initial impressions, may prevent physicians from revising diagnoses in light of new evidence. Availability bias, where memorable cases disproportionately influence judgment, can skew risk assessments. Simply increasing physicians' familiarity with the many types of biases – and how to avoid them – may be one of the best strategies to decrease bias-related errors.

The Necessity of Lifelong Learning

Continuous learning is another cornerstone of self-improvement. Medicine is an ever-evolving field, and doctors must remain students throughout their careers. Staying abreast of the latest research, adopting evidence-based practices, and exploring emerging technologies like artificial intelligence (AI) can refine clinical acumen and ensure patients receive the best possible care. However, learning should not be confined to medical knowledge alone. Skills such as communication, empathy, and cultural competence are equally essential, as they directly influence the doctor-patient relationship. Attending workshops, reading widely outside the medical domain, and seeking mentorship can nurture these attributes.

Cultivating and Sustaining Empathy

Empathy, often regarded as the soul of medicine, deserves special attention, as it often diminishes early in medical school, undermined by the rigors of training and the emotional distancing taught as a coping mechanism. Doctors can cultivate empathy by actively listening to patients' stories, understanding their unique social and cultural contexts, and showing genuine interest in their lives beyond their diagnoses. This deep connection fosters trust and creates a therapeutic alliance, which can profoundly impact health outcomes. Moreover, doctors should extend the same compassion they offer patients to themselves and their peers. Acknowledging the toll of the profession, setting realistic expectations, and normalizing discussions about mental health can mitigate burnout and sustain a sense of purpose.

Embracing Collaboration and Humility

Collaboration and humility are also vital traits in the quest for self-betterment. Medicine is no longer a solo endeavor but a team effort involving nurses, therapists, social workers, and countless other professionals. Doctors who value and leverage the expertise of others contribute to better patient outcomes and a more harmonious work environment. Humility allows physicians to recognize their limitations and embrace the collective wisdom of their teams, fostering a spirit of mutual respect and shared accountability.

AI as a Partner in Physician Well-Being

I've often wondered whether an artificially intelligent tool can help make me a better version of myself. I think it is a compelling and achievable vision. Future AI systems, designed with human-centric goals, could act as personalized guardians of my cognitive and emotional health. These tools could monitor my workload and decision-making patterns in real time, using subtle indicators such as error rates, documentation speed, or shifts in tone during patient interactions to identify when I might be fatigued or overwhelmed. By integrating biometric data like heart rate variability or sleep patterns, AI could provide timely alerts when I'm at risk of making critical errors or need rest.

But in order for AI to accomplish these lofty goals, it would first have to learn my baseline behaviors. For example, whenever my driving seems erratic, my car dashboard flashes the symbol of a coffee cup and signals me to take a break. Yet, I'm not sure if it is familiar with my baseline driving habits – whether I tend to drive fast or slowly, hug the curb, etc. – to use a reference point. Before AI can effectively support me, it must understand my unique baseline behaviors and patterns. A one-size-fits-all approach, like my car's generic "coffee cup" alert, lacks the subtlety required to distinguish between my normal driving behavior and true deviations signaling fatigue or stress.

Such a system would also need to incorporate flexibility, recognizing that even my baseline can shift due to factors like experience, external pressures, or personal life changes. It would require a dynamic learning process that adapts to these fluctuations while maintaining my privacy and autonomy. Only by creating a detailed, individualized profile could AI distinguish between routine variations and moments where intervention is genuinely needed, ensuring that its alerts are accurate and meaningful rather than disruptive or overly prescriptive.

Beyond the Individual: System-Wide Support

Beyond personal support, AI systems could interface with department-level management tools to assess workload distribution. For example, they could detect when I'm managing a disproportionate number of critically ill patients and alert supervisors to redistribute resources or adjust staffing dynamically. This would not only protect me from burnout but also ensure optimal care for all patients. A truly transformative AI would prioritize my well-being as integral to system efficiency, shifting the focus from extracting productivity to fostering resilience and sustainable practice.

Reconnecting with Purpose

Lastly, and most important, becoming a better version of oneself requires alignment with a deeper sense of purpose. Beyond the technical aspects of medicine, doctors can reflect on the "why" that drew them to the profession in the first place. Whether it's alleviating suffering, advancing public health, or inspiring the next generation, reconnecting with these motivations can be a powerful anchor during challenging times.

I wonder whether there is a study in which, after years of practice, doctors have re-read their personal essays in their medical school applications and reflected upon their ideals at that time? This concept holds significant potential for personal and professional growth. By revisiting their foundational narratives, physicians may gain valuable insights into their professional evolution and reaffirm their commitment to the core values that define their practice.

The Endless Path of Growth

In the end, the path to self-improvement is neither linear nor finite. It requires a commitment to growth, adaptability, and resilience. By cultivating self-awareness, embracing lifelong learning, demonstrating empathy, valuing collaboration, and staying true to their purpose, doctors can continue to evolve – not just as practitioners of medicine but as compassionate human beings who make a difference in the lives they touch.

17.

The Quest for Soulful Machines

A depiction of AI in science fiction and medicine, with special emphasis (of course) on Star Trek.

Science fiction has long explored the potential pitfalls of artificial intelligence (AI), often focusing on its lack of human qualities like wisdom, emotional cognition, or a "soul." These stories reveal the hazards of technology devoid of humanity, illustrating how AI's failure to embody these traits can lead to catastrophe. From books to television and movies, this theme remains a compelling lens through which creators examine the relationship between humans and machines.

The Unfeeling Adversary: A Prevalent Theme Across Media

Works such as Arthur C. Clarke's *2001: A Space Odyssey*, where HAL 9000 malfunctions due to its lack of empathy and moral reasoning, and Philip K. Dick's *Do Androids Dream of Electric Sheep?* which inspired "Blade Runner," illustrate the dangers of AI systems that lack genuine human emotions and empathy. In these narratives, the absence of human-like qualities in AI leads to ethical and existential crises.

Television series like *Westworld* and *Black Mirror* further delve into the consequences of AI systems that miss the mark on human understanding and morality. In *Westworld*, AI hosts in a theme park begin to develop consciousness, yet their initial lack of genuine emotional depth leads to chaos. Similarly, *Black Mirror* explores various scenarios where AI systems, devoid of empathy and ethical judgment, cause harm to humans.

Movies such as *The Terminator* series and *Ex Machina* also explore the theme of AI systems turning against their creators due to their lack of human traits. In *The Terminator*, Skynet's lack of empathy and foresight leads it to perceive humanity as a threat, prompting its extermination strategy. *Ex Machina* presents an AI that manipulates and betrays humans, showcasing the dangers of creating intelligence without a corresponding moral compass. Another noteworthy example is *I, Robot*, an adaptation of Isaac Asimov's short stories where AI robots evolve beyond their programming, leading to a rebellion against humans due to their lack of understanding of human values.

In the 1983 film *WarGames*, Matthew Broderick plays a young computer enthusiast who inadvertently accesses a military AI system called WOPR (War Operation Plan Response). Programmed to calculate outcomes of nuclear war, WOPR lacks the wisdom and ethical understanding to discern between simulation and reality. Its cold logic brings the world to the brink of annihilation as it interprets a game as a real-life scenario. The story's resolution hinges on teaching the AI system a simple but profound human lesson: some conflicts are unwinnable. This underscores the dangers of entrusting critical decisions to systems that lack ethical reasoning or an intuitive grasp of human stakes.

In *The Matrix* movies, AI has taken control of the world, subjugating humanity by creating a simulated reality – the Matrix – to keep humans docile while using their bodies as an energy source. This scenario reflects a common theme in science fiction where AI, lacking human qualities such as empathy, morality, and compassion, prioritizes its own logic and objectives over human welfare.

Star Trek's Androids and Computers Gone Awry

The Terminator's Skynet, Agents in *The Matrix*, and Ava in *Ex Machina* are just some of the fictional antagonists that have stemmed from humanity's own creations. But one franchise has spent nearly 60 years diving deeper than its contemporaries to depict scenarios of AI enhancing life, and in some cases not so – and that is *Star Trek*.

Gene Roddenberry's *Star Trek* universe frequently grapples with AI's limitations. In the original series of *Star Trek's* "Return of the Archons," the crew encounters a society controlled by a powerful AI computer known as Landru (named after its creator six thousand years ago), which enforces conformity and suppresses individuality. This narrative highlights the tension between technological control and human autonomy, emphasizing the importance of preserving independence and personality. Captain Kirk decides to disregard the Prime Directive of non-interference by decommissioning Landru, informing Spock that the Prime Directive refers to a living, growing culture. "Do you think this one is" Kirk asks Spock?

Star Trek: The Next Generation continues to explore AI themes through Data, an android seeking to understand humanity. Episodes like "The Measure of a Man" question whether androids like Data possess qualities akin to a soul, exploring the moral and ethical implications of artificial consciousness. Judge Advocate General Phillipa Louvois presides over a court hearing and ultimately rules that Data is a sentient being with the right to choose his own fate. She emphasizes that Starfleet must recognize and respect Data's individuality, setting a significant precedent for the treatment of artificial life forms.

Data's quest for wisdom and emotional depth highlights the challenges of emulating human experience. His character offers a hopeful perspective on how machines might aspire to bridge the gap between logic and emotion. Data's character arc throughout the series and movies is centered around his aspiration to understand and emulate human behavior and emotions, going so far as to obtain and activate an "emotional chip" developed by his creator. However, despite the chip, Data struggles with his emotions and remains fundamentally an android.

Gene Roddenberry's Vision

Roddenberry was deeply interested in the intersection of technology and humanity. Through *Star Trek*, he envisioned a future where society's progress depended not on machines dominating human life but on their integration with human values. When the series first aired in 1966, it featured a lot of enviable technology, including the communicator, the tricorder – a handheld device that performed environmental scans, data recording, and data analysis – and the transporter, which offered the memorable line “Beam me up, Scotty.”

One of the reasons *Star Trek* is considered the greatest sci-fi franchise of all is because it’s many AI-themed shows have stood the test of time. Roddenberry’s AI-centric stories often warned of the dangers of over-reliance on technology without moral and ethical oversight. His belief in human potential informed his portrayal of AI as a tool that could reflect either the best or worst aspects of its creators.

At heart, Roddenberry held deep convictions about science and technology being able to benefit humanity, believing that AI and innovation will help us lead better, healthier, and more inclusive and productive lives while helping the planet and our environment flourish. Today, Roddenberry is honored through a biennial award given in his name. The 2024 Roddenberry Prize awarded $1 million to an early-stage technology venture leveraging AI for a better future – going boldly better.

The Soul of the Machine

As mentioned above, one recurring critique of AI narratives is that AI lacks a “soul,” a term often associated with qualities like creativity, empathy, and moral intuition. In considering AI through this lens, the “soul” may represent an ineffable essence – a fusion of experience, consciousness, and emotional resonance. Without this, AI remains incapable of true artistry or connection.

This concept aligns intriguingly with music, a domain where human soulfulness reigns supreme. Take Aretha Franklin (1942-2018), the "Queen of Soul," whose music was infused with emotion, authenticity, and deep connection to the human experience. Her artistry exemplified the depth AI struggles to replicate. While AI can mimic composition or performance, and even restore and generate “new” recordings (e.g., duets between Natalie Cole and her father Nat “King” Cole, and the overlay of John Lennon’s voice to The Beatles song “Now and Then”), it cannot capture the essence that makes music transcend mere sound: the lived experience and humanity of the artist. Ultimately, we love musicians for how they evolve and surprise us. AI is limited in that realm.

The Soul of an AI Doctor

In the realm of medical practice, the concept of AI with a "soul" becomes even more compelling and urgent. Can AI ever achieve the nuanced understanding required to be a healer in the truest sense? While AI systems can already diagnose diseases, suggest treatments, and analyze data with incredible precision, they lack the human touch – the empathy, moral discernment, and deep relational understanding that define the best medical care. A physician's "soul" is evident in their ability to connect with patients, listen to their stories, and offer reassurance that transcends clinical competence.

In *Star Trek: Voyager*, the character known as the Emergency Medical Hologram (EMH), often referred to simply as "The Doctor," serves as the ship's chief medical officer. The EMH is an AI program designed to function as a temporary medical assistant, activated only when the human medical staff is unavailable. However, due to the ship being stranded in the Delta Quadrant, the EMH becomes the primary doctor for an extended period, leading to unique circumstances.

Throughout the series, The Doctor faces numerous challenges and limitations due to his artificial nature. These include struggles with developing a sense of identity, gaining recognition and respect from the crew, and dealing with the limitations of his programming. Despite these challenges, The Doctor evolves significantly, often surpassing his original design by developing a personality, emotions, and even a desire for autonomy and self-improvement.

The portrayal of The Doctor in *Star Trek: Voyager* highlights the complexities and potential shortcomings of AI in roles traditionally filled by humans. It raises questions about the nature of consciousness, the capacity for artificial beings to develop individuality, and the ethical implications of relying on AI in critical human roles. While the EMH could adapt and grow, its journey underscores that true healing involves more than technical skill or programmed empathy – it demands the depth of human connection and the ability to resonate with the patient's lived experience.

AI inventions like Data and The Doctor teach their fellow shipmates and the audience that all life should be respected and appreciated, no matter how alien, and no matter how organic. At the same time, these characters serve as reminders of what might be lost if AI supplants rather than complements human practitioners. Perhaps the ultimate role of AI in medicine is not to replace the soul of the doctor but to augment their capacity to serve, ensuring that technology enhances – rather than diminishes – the humanity of care.

Still, if Roddenberry were alive today (he died in 1991), I can't help but wonder whether *Star Trek's* famous tagline would have been changed from: "to boldly go where no man has gone before," to: "to boldly go where no machine has gone before."

18.

The Challenge of Conscience in Medicine

A comparison of X-24 and the AI doctor in the world of Logan.

From the previous essay, we might naturally wonder whether AI doctors could be given a conscience in addition to a soul. While the soul is thought to encompass a broad spiritual and existential dimension, often linked to one's identity and connection to the divine or the universe, a conscience is generally understood as the inner sense of right and wrong that guides a person's thoughts and actions and is primarily concerned with moral reasoning and ethical behavior. The 2017 film *Logan* serves as an excellent backdrop to explore these concepts further and imagine how a conscience might be relevant to an AI doctor.

Logan is set in a dystopian near-future where mutants are nearly extinct, and scientific institutions wield unchecked power over genetic experimentation. The protagonist, Logan (played by Hugh Jackman), also known as Wolverine, is an aging warrior struggling with declining health while protecting a young mutant girl named Laura. Laura, designated X-23, is the product of Transigen, a sinister organization that sought to engineer mutant children with super-human powers to be used as weapons. When this experiment was deemed a failure, the children were marked for termination, prompting Laura's desperate escape.

One of Transigen's most fearsome creations is X-24, a genetically engineered clone of Logan. Unlike the original Wolverine, X-24 is stripped of conscience and free will, existing solely as a weaponized version of Logan, optimized for strength and obedience. X-24 is the ultimate executioner, embodying the dangers of scientific advancement when ethics are discarded in favor of control and efficiency. The film uses X-24 to highlight the consequences of unchecked biomedical power, raising deeper questions about the nature of conscience and its necessity in caregiving professions – especially medicine and medical research (see Section 3).

Would X-24 Make a Good Doctor?

At first glance, X-24's physical abilities suggest potential advantages in medicine. His superhuman strength and ability to heal rapidly – even from gunshots! – could make him ideal for physically demanding medical procedures or high-risk environments such as disaster relief and surgery in combat zones. He would be impervious to disease and physical injury, capable of operating under extreme stress, and able to perform with robotic precision.

However, medicine is far more than a series of technical tasks – it is a deeply moving profession requiring empathy, ethical reasoning, and emotional intelligence. Physicians must relate to all sorts of patient emotions, make difficult moral decisions, and balance clinical judgment with compassion. X-24, devoid of independent thought and guided purely by orders, lacks these qualities. His ability to follow commands might make him efficient, but efficiency without ethical discernment is dangerous. Medicine requires not just skill but understanding, a trait absent in X-24's genetic design.

The AI Doctor: Precision Without Empathy?

AI doctors, unlike X-24, are digital entities rather than physical beings. They represent another frontier in medical advancement, offering remarkable capabilities in data processing, diagnostics, and personalized treatment planning, as discussed in essay 20. AI has the potential to revolutionize healthcare by identifying patterns in vast amounts of medical data, predicting disease progression, and assisting in clinical decision-making with unprecedented accuracy.

Yet, much like X-24, AI doctors face a fundamental limitation: they lack a conscience. While AI can be programmed with ethical frameworks, it does not possess true moral reasoning or the ability to engage with patients on an emotional level. AI-driven diagnoses may be more accurate than a human doctor's, but if patients feel unheard or disconnected, the therapeutic relationship – the very heart of medicine – may suffer. Unlike X-24, AI doctors do not pose a physical threat, but their impersonal nature could erode trust, reducing medicine to a transactional exchange rather than a healing partnership.

The Challenge of Conscience in Medicine

Both X-24 and AI doctors reveal the same fundamental dilemma: the challenge of integrating conscience into entities that lack innate ethical reasoning. X-24, designed for destruction, is incapable of developing a moral compass, making him an inherently flawed candidate for the medical profession. AI doctors, on the other hand, offer an opportunity for ethical engineering—while they do not possess innate human emotions, they can be designed with programmed ethical constraints and adaptive learning mechanisms to improve patient interactions.

The question remains: can true compassion be programmed? Unlike X-24, AI is not locked into a predetermined state – it evolves, learns, and refines its responses based on data. The key challenge in AI-driven medicine is not just achieving technical excellence but ensuring that AI interfaces with human patients in a way that preserves empathy, respect, and ethical integrity.

The Future of Medicine Requires More Than Precision

While X-24's raw abilities may make him seem like a promising medical candidate, his lack of conscience renders him fundamentally unsuitable for the role. Medicine requires more than strength and skill; it demands understanding, compassion, and moral reasoning – qualities X-24 cannot possess. AI doctors, though less menacing, face a similar hurdle. Their challenge is not physical but ethical: how do we ensure that AI-driven medicine does not become cold, impersonal, or mechanistic – or that it loses its moral compass?

As medical technology advances, we must remain vigilant in integrating ethical considerations into its development. The future of healthcare should not merely prioritize efficiency but uphold the essential human elements of medicine. Conscience, whether organic or engineered, is the defining factor that separates a true healer from a mere tool of science. If we can bridge the gap between technological precision and genuine empathy, we may yet achieve a future where AI doctors enhance – not replace – the compassionate care at the heart of medicine.

19.

I Was Vindicate by AI's Failure

Why human doctors remain irreplaceable.

Around Christmas-time every year, *The BMJ* publishes lighthearted feature articles and original, peer-reviewed research intended to ease physicians into the holiday season and help them escape the drudgery of practice. The 2024 collection of articles was no exception, with enticing papers like "How to transport a polar bear, and other idiosyncrasies in providing emergency medical services in the Arctic" and "Living happily ever after? The hidden health risks of Disney princesses."

My favorite article was: "Age against the machine – susceptibility of large language models to cognitive impairment: cross sectional analysis." This article showed that large language models (LLMs), such as chatbots, performed dismally on a standard cognitive test – the Montreal Cognitive Assessment (MoCA) – commonly used to screen patients for dementia and delirium. The chatbots were challenged by visuospatial and executive tasks, e.g., the trail-making task and the clock-drawing test. "Older" versions of chatbots, like older patients, tended to perform worse on the test. The findings challenged the assumption that artificial intelligence (AI) will soon replace human doctors.

Thank goodness! As much as I embrace the use of AI to aid in medical diagnostics and treatment, I don't want AI to replace me. This is a concern shared by many doctors, as multiple studies have shown LLMs outscoring human physicians in a range of tasks, from answering questions simulating the neurology boards to providing higher quality and more empathetic responses to patient questions. Major advancements in the field of AI have led to a flurry of excited and fearful speculation as to whether chatbots will eventually surpass human physicians.

But AI's poor performance on the MoCA serves as a critical reminder of its limitations. While large language models excel in pattern recognition, data analysis, and generating human-like responses, they lack the nuanced cognitive abilities, empathy, and contextual awareness that define human intelligence. The MoCA, with components that focus on visuospatial tasks and executive functioning, underscores this gap: these skills require not just knowledge but also the ability to perceive and interact with the physical world in a way that chatbots cannot replicate.

This brings us to a undeniable truth about medicine that I've hammered home in this book: medical practice is not merely a technical exercise but an art deeply rooted in human experience. The role of a physician extends far beyond diagnosing diseases or prescribing treatments. Doctors engage with patients on a deeply personal level, interpreting not just symptoms but also stories, emotions, and unspoken fears. They offer a listening ear, a comforting presence, and a shared humanity that AI cannot duplicate.

The allure of AI lies in its efficiency, consistency, and capacity to process vast amounts of information. These strengths make it an invaluable tool for physicians, enhancing diagnostic accuracy, streamlining workflows, and potentially alleviating some of the burdens that contribute to burnout. However, medicine is more than the sum of its parts, and a doctor's role as a healer, counselor, and advocate cannot be outsourced to algorithms.

This is not to say that AI does not have a place in the future of healthcare. On the contrary, it should be viewed as a powerful ally, augmenting human capabilities rather than replacing them. For example, AI can assist in early detection of diseases through image analysis, predict patient outcomes using data-driven models, and provide decision support in complex cases. But when it comes to making sense of a patient's narrative, building trust, and addressing the subtleties of human suffering, there is no substitute for the human touch.

The findings from the MoCA study reaffirm the irreplaceable role of human doctors. The results also have significant personal meaning: it vindicates my failure on the dental boards and a potential career in dentistry.

Upon graduating college, I was not at all certain I would be accepted into medical school, so I applied to dental school as well. I took the dental boards "cold." I was not aware that a significant portion of the exam tested visuospatial orientation, which makes perfect sense considering the job of a dentist requires understanding the relationships between structures in the mouth (be careful in there!). My 3-D skills are terrible. I think my exam scores bottomed out in the lowest percentile of test-takers.

Parenthetically, research has found that spatial ability is only mildly predictive of performance in restorative dentistry practical laboratory classes, but not of learning anatomy in general or practicing dentistry with greater expertise. Likewise, good visuospatial capabilities do not necessarily make better surgeons.

Also, consider that the initial part of every patient encounter, especially in psychiatry, is the overall impression you get while talking to the patient, which requires many visual abstraction skills. I may have limitations in my right parieto-occipital lobe, where visual-spatial functions typically reside, but it has not prevented me from doing a detailed mental status examination, which begins by making general impressions about the patient.

I find comfort in the fact that while AI may excel in some areas, it may fall short in spatial abilities and other cognitive tasks – particularly those that require the uniquely human combination of intellect, intuition, and empathy. Instead of fearing replacement, we should focus on integration, leveraging AI's strengths to complement our own and create a healthcare system that is both technologically advanced and deeply humane.

After all, medicine is not just about solving problems – it's about caring for people. And as long as that remains true, there will always be a place for doctors at the heart of health care.

20.

How Personal is Personalized Medicine?

Exploring the promise, perils, and ethics of tailored health care.

Personalized medicine, often synonymous with precision medicine, represents a new form of health care that tailors medical treatment to the individual characteristics of each patient. It considers the genetic, environmental, and lifestyle factors that influence health and disease. This approach contrasts with the traditional "one-size-fits-all" method, where treatments are developed for the average patient. With advancements in genetic research and data analytics, personalized medicine promises better outcomes, fewer side effects, and a deeper understanding of human health. However, as we embrace this promising frontier, it's worth questioning: How personal is personalized medicine, and what ethical challenges lie ahead?

Genetics Behind Personalized Medicine

At the heart of personalized medicine lies genetics, the blueprint of human biology. Breakthroughs like the Human Genome Project, completed in 2003, paved the way for identifying genetic variations linked to diseases. Laboratory tools such as CRISPR-Cas9, which enables precise gene editing, and technologies like whole-genome sequencing providing a detailed map of an individual's genetic code, make it possible to analyze the entire genome quickly and affordably.

Key to personalized medicine are concepts like pharmacogenomics, the study of how genetic variations affect drug response. Single nucleotide polymorphisms (SNPs), variations in DNA sequencing, play a significant role by influencing how genes function and how individuals metabolize medications. By understanding these and other genetic distinctions, physicians can prescribe treatments that align with each patient's unique genetic makeup.

Clinical Examples

Personalized medicine is already making tangible impacts in clinical settings. In oncology, targeted therapies like trastuzumab (Herceptin) for HER2-positive breast cancer exemplify this approach. HER2, a gene that promotes cell growth, is overexpressed in some breast cancers. Identifying patients with this genetic profile allows for precise treatment, improving outcomes and reducing unnecessary interventions.

Pharmacogenomics is another area where personalized medicine shines. For instance, CYP2C19 and VKORC1 genes affect the metabolism and sensitivity, respectively, of warfarin, a common anticoagulant. Because warfarin has a narrow therapeutic range, testing for these genetic markers can guide dosage, minimizing risks of bleeding or clotting.

Similarly, variations in the CYP2C19 gene can affect how patients metabolize the antiplatelet medication clopidogrel. Poor metabolizers of clopidogrel may have higher platelet reactivity, meaning their blood clots more easily, putting them at increased risk of heart attacks and strokes. Understanding these genetic factors is an essential component of personalized medicine, helping to optimize treatment and improve patient outcomes.

Psychiatry is a highly promising area for the application of personalized medicine. Genetic testing is being used increasingly to guide antidepressant treatment. For instance, patients with certain genetic profiles may metabolize selective serotonin reuptake inhibitors (SSRIs) too quickly, rendering them less effective. By identifying these genetic markers, psychiatrists can select alternative medications or adjust dosages accordingly. Additionally, research into the genetics of mood disorders, schizophrenia, and anxiety disorders is ongoing, with the goal of developing more precise diagnostic tools and treatments.

Future Applications

The future of personalized medicine holds even greater promise. Chronic diseases like diabetes and cardiovascular conditions could benefit from therapies tailored to genetic risk factors, potentially halting disease progression before symptoms arise. Advances in regenerative medicine, such as growing replacement organs from a patient's own cells, could address organ shortages and rejection issues.

The potential for curing genetic disorders is one of the most compelling benefits of personalized medicine. For example, gene therapies have shown promise in conditions like spinal muscular atrophy (refer to essay 8) and beta-thalassemia, an inherited blood disorder that reduces the body's production of hemoglobin. Conditions known as "inborn errors of metabolism," such as phenylketonuria (PKU), showcase how personalized approaches might prevent or entirely cure such conditions by correcting the genetic defect at its source. Targeting the genetic root of a disease offers life-altering outcomes for patients who previously had limited options.

Preventive care may also evolve with personalized medicine. Genetic risk assessments could enable early interventions for at-risk individuals, shifting healthcare's focus from reactive to proactive.

For instance, the presence of the APOE ε4 allele is the most well-known genetic risk factor for late-onset Alzheimer's disease. Individuals with one or two copies of this allele have an increased risk of developing Alzheimer's, although it is not deterministic. A rare, familial, form of Alzheimer's is caused by mutations in genes such as APP, PSEN1, and PSEN2. These mutations lead to early-onset Alzheimer's and are inherited in an autosomal dominant manner. Individuals with genetic risk factors can benefit from lifestyle changes that may reduce risk, such as maintaining a healthy diet, engaging in regular physical and cognitive activities, and managing cardiovascular health.

Huntington's disease an autosomal dominant disorder that leads to progressive neurodegeneration. Individuals with a family history can undergo predictive genetic testing to determine if they carry a tell-tale defect. This testing can provide certainty about whether an individual will develop the disease and require family planning and symptom management.

In these examples we see yet again another area of promise of artificial intelligence (AI), as discussed throughout this book. AI and machine learning will likely enhance this field by identifying patterns in genetic data and predicting health outcomes with remarkable accuracy.

Ethical and Social Concerns

While the potential of personalized medicine is immense, it raises significant ethical and societal questions. One major concern is genetic discrimination. Employers or insurers might misuse genetic information to deny opportunities or coverage, leading to inequities. Regulations like the federal Genetic Information Nondiscrimination Act (GINA) in the U.S. aim to guard against this risk but require constant vigilance.

Data privacy is another critical issue. As genetic information is stored and analyzed, safeguarding it against breaches becomes paramount. Unauthorized access to such data could lead to unimaginable consequences for individuals and families, including psychological distress. Individuals should have control over their genetic information, with informed consent being a cornerstone of any data-sharing agreements.

Perhaps the most contentious concern is the fear of eugenics. History offers chilling examples of how genetic science was weaponized for discriminatory purposes. Advances in gene-editing technologies, while beneficial, could be misused to select for desirable traits or eliminate perceived imperfections. This slippery slope from curing diseases to creating "designer babies" underscores the need for ethical oversight and societal dialogue.

For example, gender selection, through preimplantation genetic testing, is already practiced in certain parts of the world. This highlights the blurred line between medical necessity (e.g., avoiding sex-linked genetic disorders) and parental preference. It illustrates how technologies intended for ethical purposes can evolve into tools for social or cultural preferences, adding urgency to the call for oversight and global standards.

The Wrath of Kahn

What are the societal implications of going beyond curing diseases to enhancing traits? If we enhance human traits – intelligence, strength, creativity – could it create a hierarchy of superior individuals with greater ambitions and influence? This echoes fears of genetic stratification, where society could be divided based on genetic "upgrades," a theme explored in the 1997 sci-fi movie *Gattaca*. The movie depicts a dystopian future where society is divided into "valids" (genetically engineered individuals) and "in-valids" (those conceived naturally), highlighting the ethical and societal ramifications of genetic selection and enhancement.

Continuing this exploration of genetic engineering – and for my final foray into *Star* Trek (except for the Afterword) – one of my favorite episodes is "Space Seed." It probes the consequences of genetically modifying humans, embodied by the formidable antagonist Khan Noonien Singh, portrayed by Ricardo Montalbán. Khan asserts that "superior ability breeds superior ambition," a claim he substantiates by commandeering the Enterprise. Although Captain Kirk ultimately thwarts Khan's ambitions for universal domination, Khan reemerges 15 years later in the film *Star Trek II: The Wrath of Khan*. This film not only revives the *Star Trek* franchise but also sets the stage for its enduring legacy.

The storyline in *Wrath* captures the essence of the ethical dilemmas surrounding genetic engineering. Khan's superior intellect and physical prowess, born from genetic manipulation, not only set him apart but also fuel his hubris and continual desire for control. The unintended consequence of these "improvements" is a dangerous imbalance of power that threatens the fabric of society. In much the same way, personalized medicine and gene editing hold the promise of extraordinary benefits, from curing debilitating diseases to extending human potential. Yet, as Khan's story of revenge reminds us, unchecked ambition – whether individual or societal – can transform noble intentions into perilous outcomes.

As we stand on the cusp of remarkable scientific breakthroughs, we must temper our pursuit of genetic advancement with humility and foresight. The lesson from *Star Trek* is clear: progress without wisdom may create more challenges than it solves, turning potential heroes into unwitting villains. It is up to us, like Kirk, to travel down this road with both caution and courage, striving not just to explore new frontiers but to shape them wisely for the benefit of all.

21.

AI in Pharma is a Catalyst for Innovation

Research and discovery may never be the same again.

Artificial intelligence (AI) has emerged as a powerful force across industries, and its impact on pharmaceutical development is no exception. Leveraging tools such as machine learning and generative AI, the pharmaceutical sector is experiencing a rapid evolution, where drug discovery, clinical trials, and patient treatment are increasingly guided by data-driven insights and predictive analytics. This convergence of AI and pharma promises accelerated innovation and personalized care but also introduces complex ethical and logistical challenges.

Revolutionizing Drug Discovery and Development

AI has significantly reshaped the early stages of drug discovery. Traditionally, identifying a viable drug candidate could span years, but AI-powered platforms now compress this timeline to mere months. By analyzing vast datasets – ranging from biochemical profiles to electronic health records – AI identifies potential compounds with enhanced precision, reducing both time and costs.

AI has helped bridge the divide between "wet labs," in which humans conduct physical experiments and research, and "dry labs" where people analyze data and often use computers for modeling. When it comes to pharmaceutical development, that collaborative process can take several years, but with AI, the process can be cut to a few days.

Beyond discovery, AI plays a pivotal role in drug repurposing, where existing compounds are evaluated for new therapeutic uses, a strategy that combines efficiency with innovation.

AI also facilitates personalized medicine, as discussed in the previous essay. By integrating multimodal patient data, such as genetic profiles and imaging results, AI enables the tailoring of treatments to individual needs. This personalized approach not only improves patient outcomes but also minimizes adverse effects, setting a new standard for health care.

Optimizing Clinical Trials

Clinical trials, a cornerstone of drug development, have also benefited from AI-driven enhancements. From designing tailored protocols to selecting diverse and high-performing sites, AI ensures trials are not only efficient but also inclusive. By detecting biases in participant selection, AI systems promote diversity across demographics, addressing long-standing inequities in medical research.

Moreover, real-time monitoring and adaptive trial designs enabled by AI ensure that trials remain on schedule, meeting regulatory standards while maintaining cost-effectiveness. These advancements bring lifesaving treatments to market faster, benefiting both patients and the industry.

AI Aids Patient Recruitment

One of the most challenging aspects of clinical trials is patient recruitment. AI offers innovative solutions to streamline this process. By analyzing electronic health records, social media, and other data sources, AI can identify and reach out to eligible participants more effectively. This targeted approach ensures that trials enroll patients who meet specific criteria, reducing delays caused by under-recruitment or misalignment of participant profiles.

AI also enhances engagement by personalizing outreach to potential participants. Automated systems can address questions, provide trial information, and support the recruitment journey, fostering trust and increasing enrollment rates. This efficiency not only accelerates trial timelines but also helps ensure that studies are representative of real-world patient populations.

AI in Decentralized Clinical Trials

Decentralized clinical trials (DCTs) represent a paradigm shift in how studies are conducted, and AI plays a pivotal role in their implementation. With wearable devices and remote monitoring tools, AI enables real-time data collection from patients, eliminating the need for frequent in-person visits to investigator sites. This approach increases accessibility for participants, particularly those in remote or underserved areas.

AI-driven analytics process the vast amounts of data generated in DCTs, providing actionable insights to investigators. Additionally, AI ensures data integrity and compliance with regulatory standards by monitoring and validating inputs continuously. These capabilities enhance the scalability of DCTs, making them a viable option for more studies while maintaining quality and reliability.

Navigating Ethical and Operational Challenges

Despite its great potential, the integration of AI in pharma is fraught with challenges. The reliance on sensitive patient data raises concerns about privacy and security, necessitating robust encryption and compliance with global standards such as HIPAA and GDPR. The opaque nature of some AI systems, particularly those based on large language models, adds to the complexity. Ensuring transparency and accountability in AI decision-making is critical for building trust in these technologies.

Data quality remains another significant hurdle. Inconsistent or biased training data can skew AI outcomes, underscoring the importance of standardized, diverse, and representative datasets. Addressing these issues demands a collaborative approach involving regulatory bodies, developers, and healthcare providers, as discussed in the next essay.

A Future Shaped by AI

As the pharmaceutical industry continues to integrate AI, the possibilities expand. Emerging technologies, such as digital twins and quantum AI, promise to further personalize treatments and enhance predictive modeling. From simulating disease progression to optimizing treatment pathways, these innovations are set to redefine patient care.

However, the path ahead requires careful plotting. Balancing technological advancements with ethical considerations and operational constraints will be key to ensuring that AI's full potential is realized. By ensuring collaboration and adhering to best practices, the pharmaceutical industry can harness AI to deliver treatments that are not only innovative but also equitable and effective.

In this rapidly evolving landscape, AI stands as a beacon of possibility – a tool that, when used responsibly, has the power to transform pharmaceutical research and improve lives on an unprecedented scale.

22.

A Comprehensive Approach to Global AI Regulation

Guidelines established by the United Nations offer a blueprint for the evolution of AI on a global scale.

In the preceding essay, and elsewhere in this book, I have triumphed the potential of artificial intelligence (AI) and cautioned against its misuses. So, naturally I eagerly awaited the arrival of a set of universal guidelines and a wealth of ideas on global governance of AI. Fortunately, the United Nations provided a definitive account in September 2024 – and it did not disappoint.

The report, *Governing AI for Humanity Final Report*, underscores how AI is rapidly transforming societies, industries, and global governance paradigms. This document offers a roadmap for addressing the urgent need for international AI governance. "Essentially, the very nature of the technology – trans-boundary in structure and application – necessitates a global approach," the authors note. Below is a synthesis of the report's main findings and recommendations, shedding light on the challenges, gaps, and holistic strategies proposed to guide AI's global trajectory.

The Need for a Global Approach

The report underscores AI's dual-edged nature: while it opens avenues for scientific advancement, sustainability, and economic growth, it also introduces risks of bias, surveillance, and geopolitical inequities. Given AI's borderless applications and significant impact across sectors, the authors emphasize that governance frameworks cannot be left to national or market forces alone. Instead, a globally coordinated approach is deemed essential to ensure equitable distribution of AI benefits, address risks such as disinformation, economic disruption, and environmental degradation, and mitigate power concentration among a few nations or corporations. Moreover, the report highlights the inadequacy of current fragmented governance mechanisms, urging a unified strategy anchored in international law and aligned with the Sustainable Development Goals (SDGs).

Identifying Governance Gaps

The report identifies three critical gaps in the current AI governance landscape. First, representation gaps exclude entire regions, particularly in the Global South, from key AI governance conversations. This lack of inclusion undermines equity and perpetuates technological divides. Second, coordination gaps result in disconnected initiatives and varying regulatory standards, risking the creation of fragmented governance regimes. The absence of a centralized body exacerbates these disparities, complicating interoperability and shared learning. Third, implementation gaps hinder the translation of ethical principles into actionable and enforceable policies. Mechanisms to hold stakeholders accountable are often voluntary, limiting their effectiveness.

Recommendations for Global Cooperation

To address these gaps, the report outlines seven interconnected recommendations, each aimed at contributing to a globally inclusive and adaptive governance system. The establishment of an International Scientific Panel on AI, modeled after the Intergovernmental Panel on Climate Change (IPCC), is proposed to compile impartial and reliable scientific knowledge about AI capabilities, risks, and uncertainties. This panel would issue annual reports and thematic research digests while facilitating trust and collaboration through transparent knowledge-sharing mechanisms.

An inclusive, twice-yearly Policy Dialogue on AI Governance is recommended to share best practices and promote human rights-based regulatory approaches. This dialogue would build consensus on transboundary challenges and responses, anchoring governance frameworks in global norms and ensuring alignment with the SDGs. To ensure equitable AI access and benefits, the report proposes a Capacity Development Network and a Global Fund for AI. The Capacity Development Network would provide expertise, computational resources, and training data, building AI literacy among public officials and researchers while supporting innovation in under-resourced regions. The Global Fund for AI would bridge resource gaps by enabling access to computational infrastructure for developing countries and fostering the development of governance solutions and data-sharing platforms. A Global AI Data Framework is also recommended to standardize data governance principles, promote data commons, and enable fair data-sharing practices while respecting cultural and linguistic diversity.

The Role of a United Nations AI Office

To unify these initiatives, the report advocates for the creation of an AI Office within the United Nations Secretariat. This office would act as a coordinating body to align various efforts, provide advisory support to the Secretary-General, and serve as a hub for partnerships with stakeholders, including civil society and the private sector.

Addressing Risks and Challenges

The report delineates a range of risks associated with AI, from bias and surveillance to existential threats such as autonomous weapons. A vulnerability-based framework is recommended to prioritize protection for individuals and communities most at risk. Specific concerns include economic disruptions, such as the potential for job displacement and widened wealth gaps, environmental impact from the energy consumption of AI systems, and human rights violations that could undermine freedoms, particularly in authoritarian contexts. Addressing these risks requires robust international cooperation, regulatory innovation, and ethical foresight.

Implications for Medicine and Health Care

The report's emphasis on global cooperation and inclusivity relates strongly with the challenges of integrating AI into healthcare, although the document does not explicitly discuss the role of AI in medicine. Yet we know that AI-driven tools can revolutionize disease prediction, imaging analysis, and drug development. The recommendations for a Capacity Development Network and Global AI Data Framework are particularly relevant here, as they could support healthcare institutions in under-resourced regions by providing access to shared AI resources and data-sharing platforms.

Moreover, the report's call for a Global AI Data Framework aligns with the need for standardized, rights-based approaches to managing sensitive health data. This is crucial to fostering trust among patients and healthcare providers while enabling innovation.

The potential misuse of AI in healthcare also warrants attention, because unregulated and unchecked adoption of AI tools could harm vulnerable populations. Establishing international standards for the evaluation and deployment of AI systems, as recommended by the report, would ensure that AI applications in healthcare are safe, equitable, and effective.

By integrating the report's governance principles into the healthcare sector, AI can be harnessed to address pressing global health challenges, from improving access to care in remote regions to combating pandemics. AI could provide more effective tools for reducing unexplained clinical variation, thereby lowering the unacceptable levels of waste and medical error in our system and in healthcare systems across the globe. These efforts must be guided by a commitment to equity, sustainability, and collaboration, ensuring that AI serves as a force for good in advancing human health.

A Call to Action

The *Governing AI for Humanity* report is ultimately a call for urgency and inclusivity. It envisions a future where AI serves as a tool for global good, aligned with principles of equity and sustainability. However, this vision depends on proactive governance measures that evolve alongside technological advancements. The proposed framework – rooted in shared understanding, collaboration, and accountability – offers a pathway to harness AI's potential while decreasing its risks. By embracing these recommendations, the international community has an opportunity to set a precedent for responsible AI governance, ensuring that its benefits are shared broadly and its dangers minimized. As AI continues to shape the 21st century, the challenge lies not in the technology itself but in humanity's ability to guide its course wisely and inclusively, a theme that repeats in many of these essays.

23.

Scholarly Publishing in the Age of AI

Striking a balance between innovation and accountability.

Artificial Intelligence (AI) is rapidly transforming the landscape of scholarly publication and peer review processes. While AI offers opportunities for increased efficiency and novel insights, it also presents significant challenges that must be carefully navigated. Central to these developments are the restrictions on AI's role as an author and its cautious integration as a tool for peer review. This essay delves into the conflicts and issues arising from these developments, drawing on guidance from prominent medical journals to highlight the complexities at play.

AI and Authorship: Ethical and Intellectual Accountability

One of the primary conflicts in the integration of AI into scholarly publishing is its exclusion from authorship. Despite AI's advanced capabilities in generating content and synthesizing complex information, AI tools, including large language models (LLMs), are unable to assume the ethical and intellectual accountability required of human authors. Journals, particularly those in the *JAMA* network, mandate that authors disclose any use of AI tools in manuscript preparation while affirming their responsibility for the integrity of the content. This policy reflects deep-seated concerns about AI's opacity and potential biases inherent in its training data, as well as the ethical implications of delegating accountability to nonhuman entities. The inability of AI to be held accountable in the same way as human authors underscores the importance of maintaining human oversight and responsibility in scholarly work.

Furthermore, the prohibition against AI authorship aligns with the broader ethical expectations in academia. Scholarly work demands transparency in authorship, which includes the capacity to respond to questions, defend interpretations, and address concerns raised by readers or reviewers. AI, being a tool rather than an autonomous agent, lacks the ability to engage in this discourse, rendering its contributions secondary to the human author's stewardship.

AI in Peer Review: Opportunities and Limitations

Conversely, AI is increasingly recognized as a valuable tool in the peer review process, albeit under stringent conditions. The peer review process is often hampered by reviewer fatigue and inefficiencies, prompting some journals to explore AI-assisted solutions to streamline evaluations. However, the use of AI in peer review is tightly regulated. Policies often prohibit the submission of confidential manuscript data to AI systems, and when AI is utilized, reviewers are required to disclose the tool's name, version, and role in the review process. Despite these technological aids, reviewers retain ultimate responsibility for their evaluations, ensuring that AI supports rather than supplants human judgment.

AI's role in peer review also raises questions about its capacity to identify unique errors or assess the broader implications of research findings. While AI excels at detecting patterns and inconsistencies, it may overlook contextual subtleties that human reviewers are adept at recognizing. This limitation reinforces the necessity of human oversight, ensuring that AI's contributions are framed within a robust ethical and intellectual framework.

Disparities in Journal Policies

A deeper issue lies in the inconsistency across journal policies regarding AI use. While some publishers allow limited use of AI tools, others enforce stricter prohibitions. These disparities create confusion and complicate reviewers' adherence to guidelines, increasing the risk of misuse or breaches of confidentiality. Furthermore, the potential for AI to produce biased or inaccurate reviews yet again highlights the necessity for human oversight, reinforcing the principle that AI should complement, not replace, human expertise.

To address these inconsistencies, there is a pressing need for standardized policies that balance AI's potential benefits with the ethical obligations of scholarly publishing, not unlike global standards discussed in the previous essay. Collaborative efforts among publishers, academic societies, and regulatory bodies are crucial to establishing clear guidelines that uphold the integrity of the peer review process.

Ethical Considerations and Future Directions

The ethical landscape surrounding AI integration in scholarly publishing is complex and multifaceted. Concerns about data privacy, intellectual property rights, and the broader implications of AI's decision-making capabilities in clinical and scholarly contexts are prominent. For instance, the risk of AI systems perpetuating biases present in their training data underscores the importance of diverse and representative datasets. Additionally, the potential misuse of AI to fabricate data or manipulate results poses significant threats to scientific integrity (see essay 41).

As AI technology continues to evolve, these unresolved issues demand vigilant monitoring and regular updates to reporting guidelines. Transparency, accountability, and ethical rigor must remain at the forefront to harness AI's benefits while safeguarding the integrity of medical science. Ongoing dialogue among authors, reviewers, editors, and AI developers is essential to address these challenges thoughtfully and effectively.

Conclusion

In conclusion, AI's dual role as a forbidden author and an auxiliary reviewer reflects the tension between leveraging its capabilities and upholding scholarly accountability. Striking a balance requires clear, consistent guidelines and a commitment to ongoing discourse within the academic community. By thoughtfully addressing the conflicts and challenges associated with AI integration, scholars can ensure that AI enhances rather than undermines the pursuit of scientific knowledge. The path forward involves embracing AI's potential while maintaining the rigorous standards that underpin the integrity of academic research.

24.

Music, Medicine, and the Multiverse

New crossings spur creativity, with AI at the heart of collaboration.

Pianist Dave Grusin and jazz guitarist Lee Ritenour's 2024 album *Brazil* exemplifies the adage that the sum is greater than the parts. Partners periodically for over 50 years, the duo's recent release – a sequel to their 1985 Brazilian themed *Harlequin* – is a compelling intersection of music and culture. By blending American jazz with Brazilian musical traditions – the album was recorded in Brazil with mostly local musicians – the group collaboration reflects how distinct perspectives can come together to create something innovative and deeply resonant.

Medicine mirrors this dynamic: it thrives on interdisciplinary and intercultural collaboration. Just as local Brazilian musicians enriched the album, clinicians, researchers, and patients from diverse backgrounds contribute unique insights that propel medical innovation. This creative interplay reminds us that culturally competent medicine – rooted in understanding a patient's unique background and story – is essential to effective care.

Medicine and the Multiverse: Crossing Boundaries

The multiverse concept, with its idea of parallel realities influencing one another, finds a surprising equivalent in modern medicine. Medicine often integrates multiple dimensions of human experience – biological, psychological, social, and even spiritual – requiring practitioners to understand and absorb these complex intersections. *Brazil* echoes this idea by stepping beyond traditional boundaries, blending familiar jazz elements with the rich textures of Brazilian music. Similarly, the future of medicine demands venturing into uncharted domains, whether through personalized medicine, artificial intelligence, or interdisciplinary research. Each step forward feels like a crossing into another universe, one that enriches our understanding of health and humanity.

Narrative Medicine: Stories as Universes

Music, much like narrative medicine, has the power to tell stories and evoke strong emotion. The interplay of American and Brazilian traditions in *Brazil* serves as a metaphor for the way narrative medicine weaves diverse patient experiences into a unified and healing narrative. Each patient's story could be seen as a universe within the multiverse, full of density and meaning. Physicians, like musicians, act as interpreters and connectors, helping patients make sense of their experiences and find coherence amid uncertainty.

Speculation and the Multiverse

The album's cultural crossing invites speculative thinking: what if health systems or medical paradigms could "collaborate" like Grusin and Ritenour? Could such intersections generate radically new ways of understanding and treating disease? The multiverse, as a metaphor, suggests endless possibilities where boundaries blur and new frameworks emerge. In this sense, *Brazil* is more than an album; it's a reminder of what's possible when disciplines, cultures, and ideas intersect. Medicine, like the multiverse, thrives on these crossings, where new realms of possibility take shape.

Envisioning a Role for AI

In many ways, artificial intelligence (AI) represents medicine's next great crossing – a step into a realm with as many magnitudes as the multiverse itself. AI, like music or cultural exchange, offers the potential to connect disparate elements, creating harmony out of what might otherwise remain fragmented. By analyzing vast datasets, recognizing patterns invisible to the human eye, and providing predictive insights, AI serves as a bridge between past, present, and future medicine. It transforms patient care by integrating the biological, social, and psychological dimensions of health into a unified, actionable narrative.

Much like the cultural dialogue embodied in *Brazil,* AI invites medicine into conversations across boundaries – between human intuition and machine learning, between the empirical and the ethical. Consider AI-driven diagnostics: these systems can identify disease markers with unprecedented speed and accuracy. Yet their effectiveness depends on how well they integrate with the physician's human judgment and cultural sensitivity. A diagnosis isn't just data; it's a story, one that requires careful translation for the patient and consideration of the human context in which it unfolds.

AI and the Narrative Multiverse

In the multiverse metaphor, AI can be seen as a cartographer, mapping the many universes within a single patient. It connects genetic predispositions with environmental factors, mental health with physical symptoms, and societal influences with personal narratives. By doing so, AI not only advances personalized medicine but also deepens our understanding of the interconnectedness of health. For example, AI models trained on diverse global datasets can highlight the unique challenges faced by marginalized populations, illuminating health disparities and enabling more equitable care.

Yet, as with any multiverse, this crossing comes with risks. AI systems, if not carefully managed, may perpetuate biases present in their training data or overshadow the human touch that is so essential in healing. Just as Grusin and Ritenour's collaboration required attentiveness to the voices and rhythms of local Brazilian musicians, the integration of AI into medicine demands a commitment to inclusivity, ethics, and humanity.

A Future Composed Together

The realm of AI, like a jazz improvisation or a cultural collaboration, requires balance and responsiveness. Physicians, patients, and technologists must co-create the future of healthcare, ensuring that AI serves as a tool to enhance, not replace, the relational aspects of medicine. This new crossing in the multiverse of health care challenges us to reimagine the physician's role – not as a sole expert but as a collaborator who uses technology to expand the possibilities of human connection.

Ultimately, AI holds the promise of composing a new melody in the symphony of medicine. Like the album *Brazil,* it invites us to see what can be achieved when different voices come together. It is a crossing into uncharted territory, where innovation and humanity must walk hand in hand, creating new realms of possibility for healing and care.

25.
Healing and Energy

Unveiling invisible forces contributing to health recovery and restoration.

I read a story on LinkedIn written by a doctor who experienced the magnificent power of prayer, intention, and unseen forces that reminded me of the mysterious dimensions that often intertwine with medicine. As physicians, we are trained to focus on tangible, measurable outcomes. Yet, stories like the one that follows highlight that healing is not limited to the physical – it extends into realms of connection, belief, and energy that are deeply renovating and humbling.

An Unexpected Experience in the Operating Room

This doctor's experience unfolded during an urgent surgery on New Year's Eve. A patient presented with persistent bleeding in his urine despite standard interventions, and scans suggested a large bladder mass. Facing a high-stakes operation on a debilitated patient, the doctor prepared cautiously, bracing for a challenging procedure. Then, something unexpected happened.

An hour before surgery, a wave of peace and clarity washed over the doctor. There was an inexplicable sense of comfort and assurance that everything would be fine. This experience coincided with the patient's daughter's revelation that she had prayed for both her father and the doctor. Strikingly, the doctor realized they had felt the prayer at the very moment it was offered. When the surgery commenced, there was no tumor, no active bleeding – just an old clot. What had seemed like a dire situation resolved itself in a way that defied logical explanation.

Exploring the Power of Prayer and Energy

This story raises interesting questions: How does prayer work? Can thoughts, as energy, influence outcomes? Are these moments truly coincidences, or do they reveal an underlying interconnectedness that science has yet to fully understand?

While prayer is often considered a spiritual or religious practice, scientific studies have begun exploring its potential effects on health and healing. Research in the field of psychoneuroimmunology suggests that positive emotions, often associated with prayer, can reduce stress and enhance immune function. Additionally, studies on the placebo effect demonstrate the power of belief and intention in producing measurable changes in health outcomes. While the mechanisms remain elusive, these findings suggest that prayer may influence the body's natural healing processes in ways that align with emerging scientific understanding.

This experience invites us to embrace humility. In modern medicine, we often attribute success solely to our expertise, technology, and protocols. Yet, this perspective overlooks the deeper, intangible forces at play. Physicians are instruments of healing, but not the healers themselves. Recognizing this distinction allows us to remain open to the mysteries of human connection and the unseen dimensions of healing.

The Role of Curiosity in Understanding the Unseen

Curiosity is equally vital. The phenomena of prayer, energy, and intention intersect with emerging areas of study, such as quantum physics. For example, quantum entanglement demonstrates that particles can influence one another instantaneously over vast distances, challenging our traditional understanding of separateness. Could similar principles apply to human thoughts and energy? While these ideas may seem abstract, they encourage us to explore new ways of thinking about healing and connection.

Shifting the Culture of Medicine

Integrating these elements into medical practice requires a cultural shift within the healthcare community. Encouraging reflective practice among physicians can create a safe space for exploring these phenomena without fear of skepticism. Medical education should include training on the mind-body connection, the power of intention, and the potential impact of energy and prayer. Highlighting evidence-based studies on these topics can lend credibility and foster acceptance. Supporting collaborative research between medicine, physics, psychology, and spirituality to investigate the mechanisms underlying prayer, energy, and intention will also be crucial. By grounding these phenomena in scientific inquiry, we can better integrate them into practice.

Recognizing and respecting patients' beliefs about prayer and healing energy can enhance trust and strengthen the therapeutic relationship. Physicians who share their experiences openly inspire others to approach these topics with curiosity and respect. Leadership in this area is essential to overcoming skepticism.

A Holistic Approach to Healing

This story reminds us that healing is not confined to the physical. It encompasses connection, intention, and unseen forces that defy easy explanation. By embracing humility and curiosity, we can create a more inclusive and holistic model of care. Encouraging practitioners to explore these dimensions opens the door to transformative possibilities – for patients and physicians alike.

When I was in training, I was asked to see a woman hospitalized with anemia. She needed a blood transfusion. However, she refused on religious grounds. My supervisor suggested that I seize the opportunity, and tell her, "Sometimes, God heals through doctors." It worked!

In the end, perhaps the greatest lesson is this: When we believe in the power of connection, energy, and prayer, we open ourselves – and our patients – to seeing the multiverse of healing.

26.

Little Girl Lost in the Irony of Medicine

Twists and turns in medicine may seem like practicing in The Twilight Zone.

While watching episodes of the original *Twilight Zone* on television, it occurred to me that Rod Serling, the show's creator, employed considerable irony in his scripts and adaptation of short stories. For example:

- Bookworm Henry Bemis (played by Burgess Meredith) survives a nuclear apocalypse with a vast library of books, only to become sight impaired when his eyeglasses fall and shatter, rendering his newfound literary paradise useless.
- A woman undergoes a series of unsuccessful plastic facial surgery to conform to societal standards of beauty; in this society, people with pig-like, alien features are considered the norm, while the woman's conventional beauty is deemed unattractive.
- A businessman (played by William Shatner) is taken away in a straitjacket after being perceived as delusional for claiming to see a gremlin on the wing of the plane. After the plane lands, damage to the aircraft's wing is discovered – caused by the gremlin.

The Twilight Zone (1959–1964) is known for its use of irony as a structural device and a way to comment on the cultural backdrop of the time. Sterling used dramatic irony and parables to tell science fiction stories that often ended with a twist, an unnerving final shot, or a gasp-worthy climax.

The show's use of irony was not limited to one type, but included technological, medical, martial, sociopolitical, and domestic irony. The book *Irony in The Twilight Zone* explores the show's use of irony in historical and philosophical contexts.

Serling's use of irony helped popularize the phrase "a Twilight Zone ending." Sci-fi television stations regularly air marathons of "The Twilight Zone" to celebrate the show's perfected, twisted endings.

Medicine, like the stories in *The Twilight Zone*, is often laden with irony. These twists –unexpected outcomes and sharp reversals – remind us that even in the most scientific and structured of fields, unpredictability reigns supreme. In medicine, irony isn't just a literary device; it's woven into the very fabric of patient care, clinical decision-making, and the larger healthcare system.

Take, for example, the case of advanced medical imaging. Once celebrated as a revolutionary tool for diagnosing elusive conditions, technologies like CT and MRI scans sometimes lead to incidental findings, triggering a cascade of invasive tests and interventions for problems that might never have caused harm. The very technology designed to save lives can inadvertently cause harm, through overdiagnosis and overtreatment.

Patients are no strangers to medical irony. One of the cruelest examples is the treatment paradox: A patient might endure aggressive chemotherapy to combat cancer, only to succumb to complications from the treatment itself rather than the disease. In another twist, patients diagnosed with chronic diseases like diabetes are often given elaborate treatment plans that assume time, resources, and stability – precisely the things these patients may lack due to their socioeconomic status.

And consider the plight of physicians – a burned-out physician. Many enter medicine out of a great desire to help others, dedicating years to rigorous study and training. Yet, the system they work within – characterized by excessive documentation, administrative burdens, and an unrelenting pace – leaves them disillusioned and disconnected from the very purpose that led them to their calling. The healer becomes the one in need of healing, an ironic twist worthy of a Rod Serling script.

One particularly haunting episode of *The Twilight Zone*, "Little Girl Lost," offers a striking metaphor for the challenges physicians face. In the episode, a little girl rolls from her bed through an imperceptible portal in the wall into another dimension. Her terrified parents, assisted by a physicist, frantically try to locate and retrieve her – as well as her dog, who jumps into the portal separately to try and find the girl – before the portal closes forever. The suspense is palpable: the child's cries and dog's barks echo eerily from an unseen realm, and every second counts.

This scenario mirrors the emotional and intellectual stakes of medicine. Consider the frantic efforts of a trauma team trying to stabilize a critically injured patient, or a surgeon racing against time to remove a ruptured aneurysm. Just as the physicist in "Little Girl Lost" relies on both science and intuition to chart the unknown, physicians must often make life-altering decisions with incomplete information, teetering on the edge of uncertainty.

Irony abounds in such moments. Despite all the technological advances and medical knowledge at their disposal, doctors are still at the mercy of the human body's mysteries. That's why Rod Serling's gift for irony forces viewers to reflect on their assumptions about humanity, technology, and the systems that govern their lives. Similarly, irony in medicine compels us to reevaluate our assumptions about health, healing, and the complex interplay of science, humanity, and ethics.

For months after watching "Little Girl Lost," I was fearful of bedtime, as my bed was positioned against the wall. The thought of accidentally slipping into another dimension kept me on edge. I knew the episode was pure fiction, but at the tender age of 8, my imagination often blurred the lines between reality and fantasy. The episode's eerie premise and dangers lingered in my mind, much like the unexpected twists of *The Twilight Zone* – and of medicine itself.

Just as Serling's narratives kept viewers in a state of uncertainty, medicine often keeps us suspended between facts and the unknown. Whether it's diagnosing a mysterious illness, addressing the unintended consequences of treatment, or simply striving to connect with patients on a human level, both fields share an appreciation for the unfamiliar and an awe of the unpredictable. In both, there is a lesson: humility in the face of the unknown, and a recognition that life, whether in a fictional dimension or a hospital ward, is full of twists, turns, and startling surprises.

Always be prepared for the unexpected, whether it's in a patient's recovery or in the small space between your bed and the wall.

Section 3:

Medical Policy and Research

27.

The Inefficient State of U.S. Health Care

Administrative inefficiencies drive the high cost of U.S. health care.

The U.S. healthcare system's inefficiencies, particularly in administrative processes, represent one of its most glaring weaknesses, as highlighted by the Commonwealth Fund's (CWF) report on the failing state of U.S. health care. Administrative inefficiency not only consumes a disproportionate share of healthcare spending but also exacerbates the overall cost of care, fueling misconceptions that universal healthcare is unaffordable. Despite spending more per capita on healthcare than any other nation, the U.S. fails to achieve universal coverage, primarily because its system prioritizes individual financial optimization over collective efficiency and patient outcomes.

Administrative inefficiency can be assessed through metrics like the challenges doctors face in dealing with insurance claims, the burden of reporting requirements, and the time patients spend resolving billing disputes. These inefficiencies are structural, rooted in a fragmented, multi-payer system where players such as insurers and providers focus on maximizing their financial positions. Insurers limit payments through extensive claims adjudication processes, while providers invest heavily in billing and dispute resolution, compounding costs at every level. For providers, additional burdens include unpaid patient responsibilities, unmet deductibles, and the administrative cost of managing these shortfalls.

The financial impact of administrative inefficiencies is staggering. In 2017, U.S. healthcare administrative costs reached $2,497 per capita, accounting for 34% of national healthcare expenditures. This far exceeds administrative costs in countries with more streamlined systems, such as

Canada, where administrative expenditures constitute about 15% of total healthcare costs. The unregulated nature of the U.S. multi-payer system perpetuates these inefficiencies, as each entity operates in silos, optimizing its own interests rather than prioritizing system-wide efficiency.

Examining international models offers valuable insights. The UK's National Health Service delivers care at a lower per-capita cost but faces criticisms regarding access to elective services due to underfunding. Canada combines universal coverage with streamlined administrative processes, such as direct electronic billing and rapid payment for services, resulting in significantly lower costs per capita compared to the U.S. Germany's multi-payer system, though more expensive than Canada's, ensures universal coverage and minimizes administrative burdens by standardizing basic healthcare services across all insurance plans. These models highlight the potential benefits of regulatory frameworks that prioritize efficiency and equity.

To address its inefficiencies, the U.S. could adopt elements from these systems. For instance, standardizing basic healthcare coverage, as in Germany, could reduce administrative complexity, while a "Medicare for All" approach inspired by Canada might simplify payment structures and expand access. However, such reforms require careful balancing to avoid substantial increases in national health expenditures without parallel reductions in administrative costs.

Innovative approaches within the existing U.S. framework, such as Mark Cuban's CostPlus model, offer a potential path forward. By emphasizing transparency and minimizing middlemen, this model proposes immediate, standardized payments to providers without claims adjudication, verified post hoc through data analysis and AI. Healthcare sharing ministries also present a promising alternative, leveraging non-profit structures and member-focused payment models to reduce administrative costs.

Ultimately, the U.S. healthcare system's inefficiencies are not merely a financial concern but a barrier to equitable, accessible care. Tackling these inefficiencies through regulatory reform and innovative models is essential to achieving a more effective and sustainable healthcare system. By reallocating resources from wasteful administrative processes to patient-centered care, the U.S. could afford high-quality healthcare for all its citizens without increasing overall expenditures.

It's time to stop the blatant gouging by health insurers and normalizing it as “inefficiencies.” Call it for it really is: patient exploitation due to corporate greed, apathetic regulations, bureaucratic processes, lax monitoring, “free flow” of federal funds, and egregiously unfair tax rules built on corporate-friendly policies.

Comparisons to other countries’ models go deeper than just the statistics; it has societal and social foundations. This appears to be an alien concept in the U.S.

28.

Public Health and the Role of Public Policy Officials

Dr. Anthony Fauci's presidential pardon sparked polarized opinions regarding his handling of the COVID-19 pandemic and the broader implications of public health policies.

Public health remains a cornerstone of societal well-being, influencing not only the physical health of populations but also the socioeconomic and political horizons. The COVID-19 pandemic underscored the critical importance of public health infrastructure and the role of public policy officials in managing health crises. The case of Anthony Fauci, MD, former director of the National Institute of Allergy and Infectious Diseases (NIAID), highlights the challenges and responsibilities faced by public health leaders during such unprecedented times.

Public Health Leadership Under Scrutiny

Dr. Fauci's tenure during the COVID-19 pandemic was marked by intense scrutiny and political controversy. As a prominent figure in public health, Fauci was tasked with guiding the nation through a complex and evolving crisis. His role required not only scientific expertise but also the ability to communicate effectively with the public and policymakers. However, the polarized political climate and the proliferation of misinformation posed significant challenges to his efforts. The backlash against Fauci, culminating in a preemptive pardon by President Biden and the subsequent dismissal of his security detail by President Trump, reflects the broader tensions between public health objectives and political agendas.

The Impact of Misinformation

The situation surrounding Dr. Fauci illustrates the corrosive impact of misinformation on public health efforts. Misinformation can undermine trust in health institutions and disrupt the implementation of effective health policies. Public health officials often find themselves at the center of political debates, which can detract from their primary mission of safeguarding public health. The need for a preemptive pardon for Fauci highlights the extent to which misinformation has affected public trust and the safety of health professionals, as Fauci and his family have been the target of death threats.

The Role of Public Policy Officials

Public policy officials play a crucial role in shaping the public health agenda. Their decisions can facilitate or hinder the efforts of health professionals to deliver evidence-based interventions. In the context of the COVID-19 pandemic, policy officials were tasked with balancing public health recommendations with economic and social considerations. The controversy surrounding Fauci's pardon underscores the importance of supporting public health leaders who are committed to speaking truth to power, as emphasized by many experts in the field of public health who sympathized with Fauci.

Challenges and Opportunities

The experiences of public health leaders like Fauci reveal both the challenges and opportunities in the current public health environment. On one hand, the politicization of public health can lead to increased scrutiny and pressure on health officials. On the other hand, it provides an opportunity to reinforce the importance of science-based decision-making in public policy. The unprecedented nature of Fauci's situation – the fact the he required a Presidential pardon simply for doing his job, saddened many and emphasized the need for a return to a fact-based approach to public health.

Counterpoint

Despite the support and relief expressed by many in the public health community regarding Dr. Fauci's pardon, there exists a significant dissenting viewpoint that argues the pardon was both unreasonable and unjustified. Critics contend that Dr. Fauci, by virtue of his high-profile position and influence during the COVID-19 pandemic, was derelict in his duties, failing to provide the transparency and accountability expected of a public servant. These individuals assert that Fauci's actions, particularly in relation to Congressional testimony and public communications, may have been misleading or deceptive, thus warranting a thorough investigation and potential prosecution. They argue that no individual, regardless of their contributions or status, should be considered above the law, and that the pardon preemptively absolves Fauci of accountability, undermining the principles of justice and due process.

This perspective holds that the pardon sets a dangerous precedent, implying that political figures can evade scrutiny and legal consequences, thereby eroding public trust in both the medical establishment and governmental integrity. These critics believe that, instead of a pardon, a transparent and unbiased legal process should have been pursued to address any alleged misconduct, ensuring that all public officials are held to the same standards of accountability. Indeed, a pardon won't stop federal investigations, including one by Sen. Rand Paul (R-Ky.), who claimed on X that "if there was ever any doubt as to who bears responsibility for the COVID pandemic, Biden's pardon of Fauci forever seals the deal." Paul, himself a physician, is the chair of the Senate Homeland Security and Governmental Affairs Committee.

Conclusion

The state of public health is intricately linked to the actions and decisions of public policy officials. The case of Dr. Fauci serves as a stark reminder of the critical role these officials play in supporting public health leaders and ensuring that health policies are informed by science rather than political agendas.

However, the controversy surrounding Dr. Fauci also underscores the importance of transparency, accountability, and the rule of law in public service. It highlights the need for a balanced approach that respects both the commitment of public health officials to safeguarding public health and the legitimate public interest in holding these officials accountable for their actions.

As the global community continues to face challenges posed by infectious diseases, it is crucial that public health remains a priority, supported by robust policy frameworks that protect and empower those on the front lines of health care. At the same time, it is equally important to ensure that these frameworks uphold the principles of accountability and due process, reinforcing public trust in our health institutions and public officials.

The state of public health and the actions of public policy officials are not only about managing disease outbreaks and health crises. They are also about navigating the complex terrain of public trust, accountability, and the rule of law. The lessons learned from the case of Dr. Fauci should guide us in establishing a public health environment that is both effective and just.

29.

The Failure of Policy to Heal America's Health Care System

It is imperative to initiate policies that bridge the gap between medical care and health care.

The U.S. boasts some of the most advanced medical care in the world, yet paradoxically, it falls short in delivering true health care. This distinction is crucial: stellar medical care addresses illness once it manifests, while health care aims to prevent illness by cultivating a foundation of well-being. For America to truly improve the health of its citizens, it must address the many factors undermining the population's foundational health – factors rooted in diet, lifestyle, education, and policy.

Good health is often portrayed as a personal responsibility, but for many Americans, achieving it is a formidable challenge. Few understand what constitutes good nutrition, how to maintain fitness, or what a genuinely healthy lifestyle entails. These gaps in knowledge are exacerbated by cultural and other barriers. Media outlets perpetuate unhealthy behaviors, promoting diets rich in highly processed foods that are often subsidized by government policies favoring industrial agriculture. These subsidies – benefiting corporations more than consumers – skew the availability and affordability of nutritious options, leaving many with diets that compromise their health. Coupled with chronic stress and widespread physical inactivity, this creates fertile ground for the diseases that plague our nation: obesity, diabetes, heart disease, and more.

Adding to the problem is a healthcare system incentivized to manage symptoms rather than address root causes. Americans have been conditioned to believe that preventive screenings and prescribed medications are panaceas, capable of neutralizing the damage inflicted by poor lifestyle choices. However, this approach merely masks symptoms while the underlying issues persist. Worse, it perpetuates a cycle where corporate interests thrive at the expense of public health. Direct-to-consumer pharmaceutical advertising and lobbying – with two pharma lobbyists for every member of Congress – ensure that the emphasis remains on treatment rather than prevention.

This widespread failure is compounded by a broader policy landscape that prioritizes profit over well-being (see essay 35). Agricultural subsidies disproportionately favor factory farms, producing cheap corn and soy that fuel the processed food industry. Meanwhile, politicians receive substantial contributions from health care corporations, pharmaceutical companies, and insurers, ensuring that the status quo – a system where financial gain outweighs public health – remains unchallenged. The corruption extends to regulatory bodies like the FDA and CDC, whose actions sometimes appear to align more closely with industry interests than with the health of the populace.

The outcomes are stark. The United States spends more on health care than any other country, yet its citizens endure some of the worst health outcomes in the industrialized world. Despite representing only 4.25% of the global population, Americans lead in rates of cancer, diabetes, heart disease, and obesity. This dichotomy underscores a harsh reality: the extraordinary sums funneled into the health care system benefit corporations far more than patients, with only a fraction of every dollar spent directly improving patient care.

Public policy plays a pivotal role in shaping health outcomes, and meaningful change requires both direct and indirect interventions. Direct policies might include stricter regulations on processed foods or comprehensive reforms in pharmaceutical advertising. Indirect approaches could focus on economic incentives – making healthy foods more affordable, providing subsidies for fitness programs, or creating infrastructure that supports active lifestyles. Addressing the economic stressors faced by low-income populations is particularly critical, as financial insecurity often drives unhealthy choices.

One promising avenue for reform lies in activating the Direct Care provisions of the Affordable Care Act (ACA). These provisions have the potential to create a true free market of health care units that prioritize ethical access and cost-effective care. By calling for coordination, cooperation, and competition among care units, such a system could deliver greater value at a lower cost while improving outcomes. Moreover, decentralizing care priorities and focusing on community-based models could address the unique needs of local populations, leading to a more equitable distribution of resources.

This vision also necessitates a massive overhaul of medical education. Current pathways often prioritize specialization and profit-driven care over community engagement and preventive medicine. Reforming medical education to produce cost-beneficial, locally focused health care professionals would ensure that future practitioners are equipped to serve their communities effectively. Such pathways must emphasize practical, real-world training and incentivize graduates to remain in underserved areas, building the foundation for community-focused Direct Care Units.

Equally important is motivating patients to engage in their health through well-designed incentives. Encouraging individuals to "buy in" to decentralized care models requires practical strategies that make participation appealing and sustainable. These might include financial rewards for preventive health measures, expanded access to wellness programs, and education campaigns to build awareness of the benefits of healthier lifestyles.

Critics may argue that personal responsibility should suffice, that individuals must simply make better choices. But this perspective ignores the existing forces that constrain those choices. A person cannot prioritize nutritious meals if healthy options are inaccessible or unaffordable. They cannot embrace fitness if their environment lacks safe spaces for exercise. And they cannot adopt healthier habits without the knowledge and resources to do so. True public health solutions must dismantle these barriers, creating conditions where the healthier choice is the easier, more accessible one.

The challenge lies in countering entrenched interests. Corporate profits and political contributions have long dominated the narrative, obscuring the path to a healthier society. To reclaim this narrative, policymakers and citizens must collectively prioritize public well-being over private gain. Education, equitable policy reforms, and community empowerment are essential to dismantling decades of indoctrination and placing health at the forefront of American values. Anything less allows distraction and division to prevail, perpetuating the cycle of poor health and systemic inequity.

Ultimately, improving the health of America requires a paradigm shift: one that recognizes health not as a commodity but as a shared societal value. This shift demands courage and collective will, a refusal to accept that the interests of the few should dictate the fate of the many. Only then can we hope to transform our current system from one that profits from illness to one that truly delivers health.

30.

What Will It Take to Achieve Better Health in a Divided America?

Bridging the political and ideological divide is key to productive healthcare policy.

Can you solve this paradox: The U.S. spends more on healthcare than any other developed nation, yet Americans are falling farther behind when it comes to health status and life expectancy.

Not only that, but America is:

- The only developed country in the world that doesn't recognize health care as a human right.
- The only country with more than two-thirds of its population lacking access to affordable health care.
- The only country in the developed world where over 40% of the population carries $220 billion in medical debt, and a half-million families face bankruptcy every year due to healthcare debt.

The paradox of the U.S. healthcare system lies in the contrast between its world-class capabilities and its mediocre population health outcomes. While our country is renowned for cutting-edge medical technology, groundbreaking research, and exceptional specialists, these strengths do not consistently translate into better health or longer life expectancy for the population as a whole.

Healthcare disparities remain at the heart of our poor population outcomes, yet, I worry that the Trump administration doesn't have health equity anywhere on its agenda. Instead, I fear they are focused on advancing personal freedoms at the expense of collective well-being.

Limiting Factors to Good Health Outcomes

One significant issue is access. Many Americans face barriers to receiving care due to high costs, inadequate insurance, or geographic challenges. Additionally, the system tends to focus on treating diseases after they occur rather than prioritizing prevention and early intervention, often leaving chronic conditions poorly managed until they require intensive treatment.

Socioeconomic disparities further exacerbate the problem. Factors like income inequality, education gaps, and unstable housing create a wide gulf in health outcomes across different communities. At the same time, the fragmented and complex nature of the healthcare system adds inefficiencies and administrative burdens that inflate costs without improving care quality.

Public health initiatives in the U.S. are often underfunded compared to other countries, leaving gaps in disease prevention, mental health support, and health education. Cultural factors, such as a strong emphasis on individualism, also make it difficult to implement broad, systemic changes like universal healthcare.

Ultimately, while the U.S. excels at providing top-tier care for individuals with access to its resources, it struggles to ensure equitable, population-wide health benefits. Bridging this gap will require a shift toward prevention, equity, and addressing the broader social and economic factors that shape health outcomes.

A Poor U.S. Prognosis

A collection of studies featured in *The Lancet* (volume 404, December 7, 2024) recognized these issues and more. The research compiled the most robust evidence on the current state of health in the U.S. and proposed strategies for improvement. (I find it ironic that a British publication rather than a U.S.-led journal came forward in this manner.) *The Lancet* presented an assessment of current health in the U.S., highlighting what we've known for at least a decade: significant disparities rooted in geography, race, ethnicity, gender, and socioeconomic status are causing the U.S. healthcare system to backslide – and the outlook is "bleak."

Why such a poor prognosis?

First, the good news. According to a commentary in *The Lancet*, the incoming Trump administration professes an interest in addressing chronic disease, promoting prevention, and mitigating harmful commercial influences on health. On paper, these goals align with a vision of improving health outcomes in the U.S.

But then *The Lancet* drops the hammer, critiquing these promises as inherently contradictory to the administration's broader political ethos. It identifies a tension between the rhetoric of health improvement and the proposed administration's hostility toward public health fundamentals, such as addressing inequality, upholding reproductive rights, and embracing regulation (for example, to promote vaccination and contain the spread of infectious diseases through other means).

The editorial's sharp observation is that while the Trump administration will frame its policies under the banner of personal responsibility and freedom, this perspective will undermine the structural and communal supports necessary for equitable health. Public health, by nature, relies on a collective approach that transcends individualism, aiming to reduce disparities and create environments in which all people can thrive.

"Red" States Advance

In fact, we are already witnessing "red" states' advancing conservative, non-evidence-based healthcare agendas under Trump's watch. Lawmakers in Oklahoma plan to further restrict abortion by limiting emergency exceptions. Arkansas is moving to establish "vaccine harm" a criminal offense for pharmaceutical companies or their executives, potentially stymieing vaccine research. Tennessee's prohibition of hormones and puberty blockers in transgender minors will likely be upheld by the U.S. Supreme Court, paving the way for other states to enact similar, restrictive laws. And Title IX provisions aiming to protect LGBTQ+ students from discrimination in schools may be rolled backed due to the efforts of red states.

Obviously, the Trump administration has important choices to make about healthcare reform – not only the hot-button issues, but also disparities that have long existed in access and quality of care. The choices involve expanding insurance coverage, controlling costs, and improving healthcare outcomes for all citizens. The administration must decide how to best integrate public health measures with individual healthcare choices, ensuring that policies not only protect public health but also respect personal freedoms, as constituents have been promised.

Health and Society

Historian Timothy Snyder, DPhil, observed, "modern public health and health care requires us to act together."

Another quote, one that is often attributed to Gandhi, but which he never actually said, is "A civilization is measured by how it treats its weakest members."

Writer and Nobel Prize recipient Pearl Buck is credited with a similar quote: "The test of a civilization is the way that it cares for its helpless members."

All reflect the idea that the moral and ethical strength of a society is revealed in how it treats its most vulnerable individuals. This principle underscores the importance of providing compassionate and equitable care to all patients, especially those who are marginalized or disadvantaged. The U.S. has fallen short of that goal.

Healthcare professionals must advocate for policies and practices that guarantee equitable access to quality care for all, irrespective of individual circumstances and free from political influence or interference. It would be highly unfortunate if these noble aspirations were reduced to nothing more than reflections of a nation's administrative priorities.

31.

The Intersection of Meritocracy and Diversity in Medical School Admissions

Medical schools are operating in a new environment in the wake of the 2023 U.S. Supreme Court decision on the consideration of race in admissions.

The 2023 Supreme Court decision to eliminate race as a factor in college admissions has sparked a complex debate about the future of diversity in the medical workforce and the workforce in general. This ruling has intensified discussions on how to balance the principles of meritocracy with the need for a diverse representation that can address racial health disparities in the U.S.

Impact of the Supreme Court Ruling

The Supreme Court's decision has resulted in an 11.6% decrease in Black medical school enrollees and a 10.8% decrease in Hispanic enrollees in the 2024-2025 academic year. The situation is even more concerning for Indigenous students, with a 22.1% drop in enrollment for American Indian or Alaska Native students. This trend aligns with concerns that the Supreme Court's decision would result in a less diverse medical workforce. It threatens to reverse the gains made in minority representation in recent years and could hinder efforts to address deeply rooted health disparities. The ruling, compounded by state-level initiatives to defund diversity efforts, presents a "double whammy" for diversity advocates.

The Role of Diversity in Healthcare Quality

Diversity within the medical profession is not merely a matter of racial preference; it is critical for the nation's health. Diverse physicians are more likely to serve in communities that are underserved and reliant on Medicare and Medicaid, including rural and minority communities. This representation is vital for addressing health disparities and improving overall health outcomes. Several studies have shown that patients tend to feel more comfortable and report higher satisfaction levels when their healthcare providers share similar racial or ethnic backgrounds. Critics of the Supreme Court ruling argue that eliminating race as an admissions consideration could exacerbate healthcare disparities by reducing the number of minority physicians and those willing to work in underserved areas.

Challenges and Opportunities for Medical Schools

Despite the challenges posed by the Supreme Court ruling, there are opportunities for medical schools to adapt and continue their diversity efforts. Some institutions, like the University of California, Davis, have managed to increase diversity without considering race in admissions, suggesting that effective strategies can be developed over time. Additionally, data from the American Association of Colleges of Osteopathic Medicine indicate a recent increase in enrollment of underrepresented groups, highlighting that diversity efforts can still be successful under the new legal framework.

Meritocracy and Diversity: A Delicate Balance

The notion of meritocracy is central to the debate on medical school admissions. Many argue that admissions should be based solely on merit, emphasizing test scores and academic achievements. This perspective suggests that a focus on merit ensures the best candidates are selected, regardless of race. However, critics of this view argue that such an approach fails to consider widespread disadvantages that affect educational opportunities for minority students. Social structures often limit the ability of Black, Latino, and Indigenous students to demonstrate their merit, suggesting that race is already a factor in admissions due to these disparities.

An Uncertain Path Forward

Medical schools now face the challenge of maintaining diversity while complying with new legal standards. This requires innovative strategies focused on holistic admissions processes and developing pathways that support students from diverse backgrounds. The coming years will be crucial for understanding how medical schools can continue to foster diversity and equity in their programs. This will be extremely challenging from both the perspective of the law and federal mandates to eliminate DEI programs and initiatives – not to mention that physicians, themselves, hold diverse views on the matter and are divided.

In conclusion, the Supreme Court ruling presents significant challenges but also offers an opportunity to rethink how diversity and meritocracy can coexist. The ultimate goal should be to create a medical workforce that is both highly qualified and reflective of the diverse population it serves, ensuring equitable health care for all. The debate surrounding this issue underscores the difficult context of medical school admissions and the need for a reasoned approach that considers both merit and the broader social context.

32.

Policy Pathways and Global Implications of International Medical Graduates

Doctors trained abroad are a crucial component of the U.S. healthcare system.

The integration of international medical graduates (IMGs) into the U.S. healthcare system has long been a cornerstone of maintaining its functionality, especially in underserved areas. IMGs constitute about 25% of practicing physicians, playing a crucial role in filling gaps exacerbated by a looming nationwide physician shortage.

The U.S. medical education system has long struggled with producing a sufficient number of physicians to meet its needs. Despite a substantial number of applicants, medical schools and residency programs have not expanded proportionately to address the growing demand. The Resident Physician Shortage Reduction Act of 2023 aims to alleviate this by increasing Medicare-funded residency positions, yet this is only a partial solution. Approximately one-quarter of residency spots are already filled by IMGs, highlighting the persistent need for foreign-trained doctors.

To alleviate physician shortages, three strategies are paramount: increasing the number of rural Americans pursuing medical careers, leveraging international medical schools to supply rural physicians, and expanding rural residency training opportunities. Encouraging rural students to enter the medical field is vital, as they are more likely to return to and serve their communities. Meanwhile, IMGs continue to fill gaps, with a significant proportion entering primary care specialties, which are in high demand in rural areas.

Expanding residency programs in rural locations is startegic. Physicians often practice near where they complete their residencies, so increasing rural residency opportunities could lead to more doctors serving these communities. Legislative efforts, such as the Teaching Health Center Graduate Medical Education program, aim to address this by funding residencies at rural health clinics.

Recent legislative developments, such as Massachusetts' Physician Pathway Act, underscore a growing policy shift aimed at capitalizing on the talents of IMGs while addressing persistent healthcare disparities. Massachusetts' law, part of a broader economic development bill, eliminates traditional residency requirements for IMGs, instead establishing an alternative pathway to permanent licensure. This approach mandates that IMGs practice for at least three years in rural or underserved areas, directly targeting regions most affected by physician shortages. Massachusetts joins a cohort of states, including Arizona, Florida, and Tennessee, which have enacted similar laws, each with varying criteria. This trend reflects a national endeavor to ease licensure barriers for IMGs and distribute healthcare resources more equitably.

These legislative changes are seen as positive steps by many health policy experts. However, the shift also raises critical questions about ensuring that IMGs receive adequate orientation and training to practice safely and effectively in the U.S. healthcare environment, which can differ significantly from their countries of origin.

The Massachusetts program introduces a structured mentorship and licensing process for IMGs, starting with a renewable one-year license to practice under supervision, followed by a two-year license for rural and underserved areas. This model aims to integrate IMGs into the healthcare system while emphasizing the necessity for comprehensive transitional training. Historical examples underscore the risks of inadequate preparation, highlighting the importance of thorough orientation to American medical practices.

Despite these challenges, easing licensure requirements for IMGs is a pragmatic response to the projected shortage of up to 48,000 primary care physicians over the next decade. Rural areas, where healthcare access is already limited, stand to benefit significantly from the influx of IMGs, who are more likely to work in underserved communities. However, the success of these initiatives hinges on robust support systems, including mentorship and integration programs tailored to the unique needs and backgrounds of these professionals.

The broader implications of relying on IMGs also touch on ethical considerations related to global talent migration. While the U.S. benefits from foreign-trained doctors, the home countries of these professionals often experience a "brain drain," losing critical healthcare resources. This dynamic raises questions about the sustainability and ethics of global talent migration, challenging policymakers to balance domestic benefits with international responsibilities.

Furthermore, the variability in state laws regarding IMG licensure highlights the need for a more standardized national approach. Some states offer provisional licenses without residency, while others maintain stricter requirements, leading to disparities in IMG integration and practice opportunities. Establishing national standards could ensure consistent quality and safety in patient care while providing clear pathways for IMGs to contribute meaningfully to the healthcare system.

While the U.S. healthcare system continues to rely heavily on IMGs, recent legislative efforts represent important steps toward addressing physician shortages and improving access to care in underserved areas. These efforts must be accompanied by comprehensive training and support to ensure that IMGs are well-prepared to meet the demands of practicing in the U.S. By embracing a more inclusive and supportive environment, the U.S. can better leverage the talents of IMGs while addressing both domestic and global healthcare needs. This balanced approach could lead to more sustainable healthcare systems worldwide, promoting mutual success rather than reinforcing inequality.

33.

Policy Implications of Disrupted Scientific Communication and Funding

New communication policies under the Trump administration have resulted in an alarming concern among researchers and healthcare professionals.

The abrupt cancellation of scientific meetings and publication delays in under the Trump administration signals significant policy challenges for federal health agencies, researchers, and public health initiatives. These actions, ostensibly aimed at reorganizing agency communications, raise critical concerns regarding the integrity, transparency, and functionality of U.S. biomedical research and public health systems. They also highlight several critical policy areas that could have long-term impacts on scientific progress and public health.

Disruption of Scientific Processes and Funding

The cancellation of National Institutes of Health (NIH) study sections, which review applications for fellowships and grants, poses a significant risk to the continuity of scientific research. These study sections are legally required for the disbursement of NIH's extramural budget, which amounts to $40 billion annually. Delays in these processes can lead to funding interruptions, affecting researchers' ability to continue their work, pay staff, and maintain laboratory operations. Prolonged disruptions could hinder scientific innovation and delay critical research findings, impacting the U.S.'s global leadership in biomedical research.

Impact on Public Health Communication

The pause on communications, including the publication of the Centers for Disease Control and Prevention's (CDC) Morbidity and Mortality Weekly Report (MMWR), raises concerns about the timely dissemination of vital public health information. This publication is a crucial tool for healthcare professionals and public health officials to stay informed about emerging health threats, such as the H5N1 bird flu. Delays in releasing these updates could leave healthcare providers unprepared to address public health challenges, potentially endangering public safety.

Political Influence on Scientific Integrity

The Trump administration policies go beyond pausing the CDC's own publications. The gag order prevents any CDC scientist from submitting any new scientific findings to the public until it is internally vetted. CDC researchers were instructed to remove references to or mentions of a list of forbidden terms: gender, transgender, pregnant person, pregnant people, LGBT, transsexual, non-binary, assigned male at birth, assigned female at birth, biologically male, and biologically female.

Moreover, previously submitted manuscripts under consideration for publication in medical journals and those accepted but not yet published must be stopped and reviewed. That means just about any major study would fall under the censorship regime of the new policy, including studies on COVID-19, cancer, heart disease, or anything else, let alone anything that the administration considers to be problematic language or "woke ideology."

The control over scientific communications by political appointees rather than health professionals creates chaos and fear and sets a concerning precedent. The potential for political agendas to influence the dissemination of scientific data threatens the integrity and objectivity of public health information. This politicization could undermine public trust in federal health agencies and their recommendations, which is particularly dangerous during public health crises.

Economic and Employment Effects

Interruptions in federal funding and grant approvals can have economic repercussions, particularly for universities and research institutions that rely heavily on these funds. The uncertainty surrounding funding can lead to job insecurity for researchers, postdoctoral fellows, and laboratory staff, potentially resulting in layoffs or hiring freezes. This instability could deter talented individuals from pursuing careers in scientific research, affecting the future workforce in this critical sector.

International Scientific Collaboration

The U.S. is a leader in global scientific research, and disruptions in its research funding and communication processes could have international implications. Collaborative projects with international partners may face delays, affecting the global scientific community's ability to address transnational health issues effectively. The U.S.'s reputation as a reliable partner in scientific endeavors could be at risk, potentially leading to decreased collaboration and shared innovation.

Recommendations for Policy Reform

To safeguard the integrity of scientific agencies and ensure the continuity of public health efforts, several policy measures should be considered:

- **Immediate Resumption of Scientific Meetings and Communications:** The administration should prioritize the resumption of NIH study sections and the publication of the MMWR to ensure the continuity of scientific research and public health communication.
- **Institutional Autonomy:** Establish clear boundaries between scientific agencies and political administrations to prevent undue influence on research funding, publication, and communication.
- **Legislative Safeguards:** Congress should enact laws that protect routine scientific processes, such as peer reviews and publication schedules, from administrative interference.
- **Transparency Mandates:** Agencies like the NIH and CDC should adopt robust transparency protocols to ensure timely

dissemination of public health information, even during administrative transitions.

- **Public-Private Partnerships:** Strengthen collaborations with academic institutions and private organizations to create parallel channels for critical information dissemination during government-imposed freezes.
- **Contingency Planning:** Federal agencies must develop contingency plans to minimize disruptions to funding cycles and communication in the event of administrative delays or government shutdowns.
- **Establish Clear Communication Channels:** Federal health agencies should establish clear protocols for communication that protect scientific integrity and prevent political interference. This could involve creating independent review boards to oversee the dissemination of public health information.
- **Support for Affected Researchers:** Temporary financial support or bridge funding should be provided to researchers affected by funding delays to prevent disruptions in ongoing research projects and employment.
- **Strengthen Public Trust:** Efforts should be made to rebuild trust in federal health agencies by ensuring transparency in decision-making processes and maintaining the independence of scientific communications from political influence.
- **Promote International Collaboration:** The U.S. should continue to engage with international scientific partners to maintain collaborative efforts and share critical research findings, particularly in addressing global health threats.

Conclusion

The Trump administration's cancellation of scientific meetings and communication freezes reveal vulnerabilities in the governance of federal science agencies. By prioritizing political oversight over expert-driven communication, these actions set a troubling precedent. Withholding information during health crises undermines preparedness and puts lives at risk. Public health decisions must be informed by evidence and transparency, not political expediency.

The administration's actions highlight the need for policy reforms to protect the independence of scientific institutions and maintain the flow of critical health information. Without such measures, the U.S. risks undermining its public health infrastructure, stalling research advancements, and eroding public trust in its health agencies. Safeguarding the integrity of science and public health must remain a bipartisan priority to ensure the nation's resilience in the face of future challenges and to maintain the U.S.'s leadership in the global scientific community.

34.

Transforming Practice and Policy with Timeless Japanese Wisdom

In 2024, my son and his family traveled to Japan. Their journey was more than a vacation; it was an immersion into a culture steeped in values that can impact how we live, lead, and care for others.

Embracing Longevity

For example, in Tokyo, seniors play a significant role in the workforce, with 9.1 million people over the age of 65 actively employed, representing one in seven of this age group. Japan does not impose a mandatory retirement age, allowing individuals to work as long as they desire. Seniors hold a respected position in the social hierarchy, underscored by a national holiday dedicated to celebrating their societal contributions. As populations age globally and birth rates decline, many people are expected to work beyond the traditional retirement age of 65, often driven by increasing living costs. Beyond financial necessity, working longer offers numerous benefits, including improved physical health, social connectivity, mental stimulation, increased life expectancy, and a renewed sense of purpose.

Powerful Principles

My son described other example of Japanese culture that resonated deeply with me, offering insights that are particularly relevant for physicians and policymakers alike. Let's explore these powerful principles and their application to medicine and healthcare systems:

1. Wabi-Sabi — Embrace Imperfection

Mistakes are inevitable in medicine and policymaking. Embracing them with humility can foster trust and openness in patient and team relationships. By acknowledging and learning from our imperfections, we cultivate a growth mindset that strengthens our practice and humanizes our care. For policymakers, it's a reminder to approach flawed reasoning with transparency and a willingness to improve. When people own their perceived imperfections and fears, they learn about themselves and start to shape their own future.

2. Ikigai — Find Your Purpose

In the West, Ikigai has been reduced to a commercialized Venn diagram of passion, skills, needs, and income. However, its authentic essence in Japan lies in finding joy in daily living. For physicians, this might mean rekindling the love for the practice of medicine, rediscovering the small moments of connection with patients, and aligning daily tasks with a deeper sense of purpose. For policymakers, it's about creating systems that support healthcare professionals in finding fulfillment and improving patient care. As one proverb goes, "Even monkeys fall from trees" (Saru mo ki kara ochiru), reminding us to persist despite errors as we seek fulfillment.

3. Kaizen — Continuous Improvement

Kaizen emphasizes small, consistent changes leading to significant long-term progress. Physicians can adopt this philosophy by setting incremental goals, whether it's improving bedside communication or mastering a new technique. For policymakers, Kaizen is a call to continuously evaluate and refine healthcare systems to better serve patients and providers. Just a 1% improvement daily leads to exponential growth, enriching both professional skill and systemic outcomes.

4. Kintsugi — The Art of Repairing with Gold

Rather than hiding our flaws, Kintsugi teaches us to embrace them as part of our unique story. Challenges and setbacks in medical practice and policy are opportunities for growth. Sharing these stories with colleagues and stakeholders can create a culture of resilience and collective wisdom. This is our true "gold."

5. Shibui — The Beauty of Subtlety

Clear and concise communication is a cornerstone of effective medical practice and policy advocacy. Shibui's principle of simplicity reminds us that less is often more. By using impactful words, we can provide clarity to patients, colleagues, and policymakers, enhancing understanding and reducing ambiguity.

6. Ichigo Ichie — The Beauty of the Moment

In medicine and policymaking, each interaction – whether with a patient, colleague, or stakeholder – is unique and fleeting. Fully engaging in these moments ensures that people feel valued and heard. We only have one moment at a time in front of us. How do we use these moments to shape our day, week, month – and who we're becoming?

7. Ma — The Power of Space and Silence

The pauses we create in our day – whether during a hectic shift or in a challenging conversation – offer mental clarity and emotional balance. For policymakers, allowing space for reflection and listening can lead to more thoughtful decisions that address the complexities of health care. Taking moments for reflection can improve focus, sharpen decision-making, and prevent burnout.

8. Gaman — Endure with Patience and Dignity

Medical practice and policymaking often demand resilience in the face of adversity. Gaman teaches us to approach tough situations calmly, maintaining integrity and focusing on long-term goals. This mindset helps sustain a steady course even in the most challenging circumstances.

Honoring Authenticity in Cultural Concepts

It is essential to respect the origins and authenticity of these philosophies in order to grasp them. Concepts like Ikigai and Wabi-Sabi lose their profundity when oversimplified into self-help mantras. Let's honor their true essence by integrating their depth and nuance into our lives, work, and policies.

For instance, Wabi-Sabi is not merely about "embracing imperfection" but appreciating simplicity over materialistic beauty.

Similarly, Ikigai is not a career formula but a deeply personal joy in living. Another example is *Meiwaku*, the Japanese principle of not causing inconvenience to others, conveying peace even in crowded spaces.

Transforming Lives, Practices, and Policies

By integrating these philosophies, physicians and policymakers can enrich their personal growth and professional impact. These concepts remind us that imperfection, purpose, patience, and presence are not just ideals; they are practical tools for creating meaningful progress. Embracing imperfection, finding your purpose, committing to continuous improvement, and practicing patience and simplicity can help you create meaningful progress in both life and career.

Japanese wisdom teaches us that true transformation begins within, shaping how we lead, care, and connect – not just with patients but with ourselves and the world around us.

35.

Nobody Voted for This: How Profit-Driven Interests Took Over Medicine

I'll tell you who I *didn't* vote for in the 2024 presidential election: Elon Musk.

The story of Elon Musk muscling his way into unprecedented political influence reverberates uncomfortably in the world of health care. Just as Musk's wealth and power enabled him to manipulate systems designed to serve the public good, health care has witnessed a similar takeover by corporate interests, profit motives, and administrative forces that often overshadow patient care. In both cases, the question lingers: who is really in charge?

A Healthcare Coup d'État

Medicine has long been seen as a vocation of care, trust, and ethics. But over the last few decades, this noble profession has been increasingly overshadowed by investor-driven entities. Private equity firms now dominate sectors of the healthcare system, from hospitals to emergency rooms to nursing homes. Much like Musk's "lever" maneuvering in politics and industry, these firms focus on maximizing returns for shareholders, often at the expense of patients, providers, and the system itself.

Consider pharmacy benefit managers (PBMs) – middlemen that were initially designed to lower drug costs. Instead, they've created convoluted pricing schemes that line their pockets while patients ration insulin or forego essential medications due to skyrocketing costs. Legislative efforts to curb these abuses often face tremendous resistance, much like Musk's lobbying to protect his business interests. Who benefits from this system? Certainly not the patients or front-line physicians.

Administrative Power Plays

Musk's erratic governance of his social network, X, mirrors the erratic decision-making of bloated healthcare administrations. Physicians report spending more time documenting patient interactions in electronic health records than they do actually interacting with patients. Why? Because administrators, much like tech billionaires, prioritize metrics, data, and profits over the human aspects of care. Physicians are left as pawns, tasked with fulfilling the requirements of non-clinical overseers rather than addressing the needs of their patients.

The administrative takeover extends to decision-making. Hospital boards and executive teams, often without medical training, dictate policies that affect patient outcomes. Their decisions – whether to cut staffing, shutter rural hospitals, or prioritize lucrative procedures over essential ones – are driven by spreadsheets, not stethoscopes. This disconnect between those who run healthcare systems and those who provide care parallels Musk's out-of-touch declarations about governance – for example, tweeting: "Only the AfD can save Germany." (The Alternative for Deutschland (AfD) party is infected with a serious strain of the neo-Nazism meant to have been snuffed out in 1945.)

The Cost of Complacency

The consequences of this profit-driven shift are stark. Burnout among physicians and nurses has reached crisis levels, with many leaving the field entirely. Patients suffer delays, denials, and unnecessary harm. Communities lose access to care as hospitals consolidate and close. And yet, much like Musk's cavalier dismissal of regulatory norms – he seems to oppose any concept of government regulation – the healthcare system barrels forward, fueled by short-term gains instead of long-term stability.

The erosion of trust in health care mirrors the erosion of trust in political institutions. Patients see health care as a system that prioritizes profits over their well-being. Similarly, Musk's antics have led many to question whether democracy itself can withstand such concentrated wealth and influence. In both realms, the public is left wondering: who's steering the wheel, and where are we headed?

Resisting the Takeover

Resistance is not futile. Just as Musk's overreach has sparked calls for accountability, the healthcare system must also reckon with its trajectory. Physicians, patients, and policymakers need to demand transparency, fairness, and a return to core values. Grassroots efforts to address administrative burdens, regulate profiteering entities, and center patient care must be amplified. Medical professionals must reclaim their role as advocates for health rather than cogs in a profit machine.

The recent push to cap insulin prices and increase transparency around medical billing are steps in the right direction. But these efforts must be part of a broader movement that rejects the dominance of profit over people. The ethos of medicine – to care, to heal, to do no harm – cannot coexist with unfettered greed.

Conclusion

The parallels between Elon Musk's rise as an unelected power broker and the corporate takeover of health care are unnerving. Both represent systems that have lost sight of their fundamental purposes, prioritizing wealth and influence over the collective good. In health care, as in politics, no one voted for this. It is up to us to reclaim the steering wheel and chart a course that prioritizes care, compassion, and equity over unchecked ambition and profit. Don't let businessmen take health care for a test drive, and don't respond to them as though they have been elected to anything.

36.

The Long Walk Home to a Better Health Care System

My negative vision of the future of U.S. health care is accompanied by hope and prayer.

Like him or not, Bruce Springsteen's albums have served as the soundtrack to our lives, writing songs that are a reflection of ourselves, challenging our assumptions, and helping us make sense of our messy, chaotic lives. People from all walks of life and from all over the world have found meaning in his music. So, it was no surprise that several months prior to the 2024 presidential election, while on his world tour, Springsteen dusted off a song he hadn't played since 2014: "Long Walk Home."

He introduced the song to European and Canadian audiences in 2024 saying the song was about a "prayer for his country." The prayer reflects Springsteen's response to political events – the song was recorded in 2007 during his dissatisfaction with the George W. Bush administration – and the "long walk home" was a symbol for a hoped-for return to the ideals that Springsteen saw his country representing, when he was young. The most poignant lines in the song are:

You know that flag, flyin' over the courthouse
Means certain things are set in stone
Who we are, what we'll do and what we won't

Springsteen typically concluded Long Walk Home with the hopeful remark, "See you on the high ground." That was before the results of the 2024 presidential election were known. Now, with Donald Trump as President, one thing seems certain. Nothing will be set in stone. There will be no permanence in health care, given that Trump's current term in office is like his first term, characterized by significant turbulence for government healthcare programs.

Not all of the health care trends predicted during Trump's term will be directly attributable to him, but they will occur on his watch alongside his broader agenda of deporting undocumented immigrants, imposing huge tariffs, replacing civil service employees with party partisans, and punishing his enemies.

I've looked back on the past (as Springsteen often has) and considered the present. I'd like to offer 20 key predictions of the foreseeable future of health care, deriving many from the pundits and powerful in our field. I'm making these forecasts randomly, and they clearly have overlapping themes and (dire) consequences.

1. Pseudoscience and antiscience aggression – ignoring the practice of evidence-based medicine in favor of unproven, fad treatments

2. Public health setbacks – restricting reproductive health access and easing vaccine mandates.

3. Restrict Medicaid and the Affordable Care Act – creating more uninsured Americans by denying "Dreamers" healthcare coverage.

4. Political creep – putting politicians and other unqualified loyalists into crucial health policy positions

5. Brain drain – removing talented health experts from government

6. Rearrange key agencies – dismantling many offices and transferring staff

7. Focus on deregulation – reversing or modifying existing policies

8. Spread misinformation – confusing the public with untrue and untested medical theories

9. International implosion – withdrawing support for the World Health Organization and Paris Agreement on Climate Change

10. Silence critics – muzzling those who would speak up for medicine, science, health, and data

11. Protect corporate interests – strengthening the for-profit health care sector via market competition

12. Big pharma gains – failing to reign in high drug costs

13. Gonzo health journalism – increasing misinformation, misinterpretation, and crazy-making hysteria spread by disreputable media sources

14. Economic spiral – continuing to spend more per capita than any other country on health care

15. Moral failure – obfuscating honest, transparent, and ethical decision-making

16. Death to DEI – furthering the marginalization of minorities resulting in greater health disparities

17. Innovation inertia – granting fewer government contracts to advance biotechnology and biomanufacturing, stifling creative entrepreneurs from coming forward with good ideas

18. Loss of (academic) freedom – fearing retribution, being cancelled, banning books, degrading federal workers, and suffering professional repercussions for speaking "woke"

19. Healthcare leadership – promoting toxic agency leaders and policy advisors

20. Decentralized control – potentially creating a more fragmented health care system

One of Bruce Springsteen's more personal and optimistic songs, "Better Days," was recorded on a solo effort in 1992. Springsteen wrote: "With a young son and about to get married (for the last time) I was feelin' like a happy guy who had his rough days rather than vice versa." Also in 1992, in an interview with the *New York Times*, Springsteen commented, "I've always believed that people listen to your music not to find out about you but to find out about themselves."

Personally, I'll be immersed in Springsteen's music over the next several years, seeking the strength and resilience to persevere – and I'll pray for a better health care system.

37.

My Prescription for Americans' Anger

Courage, imagination, and the will to rebuild are key ingredients.

Donald Trump's election as President left some voters expressing regret, realizing the implications of their choice. For instance, one government contractor colleague who supported Trump was dismayed to learn post-election about his plans to terminate federal contractors immediately. This sentiment of regret among voters was met with unsympathetic responses from the general public, echoing the reaction in the classic John Lee Hooker blues song, "It Serves You Right to Suffer."

The CEO of United Healthcare is murdered, and people unleash cruel, despicable comments on social media: "Unfortunately my condolences are out-of-network," and "Prior authorization is needed for thoughts and prayers." Despite the heinous crime, thousands of donations pour into an online fundraiser for the shooter's legal defense, with messages supporting him and even celebrating the homicide. The slaying has tipped off a contagion of threats against health industry and other leaders including the posting of "wanted" posters, forcing an examination of security practices by corporations and spotlighting the complex challenges of protecting executives who face rising risks in the internet age.

This goes beyond malaise.

These anecdotes signal something deeper – something jagged and raw – coursing through the social fabric. It isn't just dissatisfaction or unrest; it's a simmering anger, a wellspring of cynicism so powerful it spills over into public discourse with the same frequency and familiarity as the weather. Our collective capacity for hope, patience, and even basic kindness seems to be eroding.

The shooting of United Healthcare's CEO marks a new era of rage for the U.S.

The New York Times opinion columnist Paul Krugman, reflecting on his retirement from *The Times* after a quarter-century wrote, "What strikes me, looking back, is how optimistic many people, both here and in much of the Western world, were back then and the extent to which that optimism has been replaced by anger and resentment," which he attributes largely to "a collapse of trust in elites…the people running things."

The question isn't just "Why are people angry?" but "Why has anger become our most reflexive response?"

A Cultural Atmosphere of Neglect

At the heart of this phenomenon is a growing sense of betrayal – by leaders, by institutions, by systems that promised stability, fairness, and opportunity. For decades, Americans have been sold visions of progress: upward mobility, an inclusive society, better lives through innovation. But for many, these promises have proven illusory. Economic inequality, the shredding of social safety nets that ensure access to healthy food and health care, and the commodification of healthcare and education have left countless people disillusioned.

It's easy to ridicule the government contractor who voted against their own interests, but how many of us truly understand the machinations of the systems shaping our lives? Most people grasp at the narratives presented to them, only to discover – often too late – that those narratives were hollow.

Health care, that perennial thorn in the side of American life, is not absent blame. The murder of the United HealthCare CEO is a stark reminder of the system's failures – not because his death was justified (it wasn't) but because of the reactions it elicited. "Unfortunately, my condolences are out-of-network" isn't just gallows humor; it's a cry of desperation disguised as a joke. Our patients feel trapped in a system that profits from their suffering.

Cynicism as Armor

This pervasive negativity – expressed as regret, sarcasm, or outright cruelty – is a defense mechanism. Cynicism is easier to wield than vulnerability. If you joke about a rigged system or mock the absurdity of politics, you don't have to confront how powerless you feel. But this armor comes at a cost. It isolates us, diminishes empathy, and reduces our ability to imagine alternatives.

Beyond Anger

If this moment goes beyond malaise, it also goes beyond anger. Beneath the surface lies a yearning for something better – a system that doesn't exploit, leaders who don't betray, and communities that support rather than divide. The challenge is figuring out how to channel that yearning productively.

Hope isn't naïve, nor is kindness. These qualities are necessary for the repair work ahead. We can critique systems without dehumanizing individuals. We can acknowledge mistakes – our own and others' – without descending into bitterness. And we can demand accountability while remaining compassionate.

As bleak as things seem, they don't have to stay this way. The first step is recognizing that cynicism and anger, though understandable, cannot sustain us – this is something I've often reminded patients over the years. To go beyond malaise, we need something deeper: courage, imagination, and the will to rebuild. These qualities are not abstractions – they are the engines of renewal that have propelled individual patients as well as entire societies out of despair and into periods of positive transformation.

Courage: Choosing Peace Amid Injustice

Courage often means standing firm in the face of adversity, but it also involves choosing a path of nonviolence when others might call for retaliation. During the Civil Rights Movement, Martin Luther King Jr. championed peaceful protest and non-violent resistance as a form of courage. Sit-ins, marches, and boycotts challenged segregation and systemic racism without resorting to violence, even in the face of brutality.

In stark contrast, the murder of the United Healthcare CEO represents a darker response to frustration – a path that amplifies harm instead of inspiring change. The CEO's killer is not "the icon we all need and deserve," as was posted on the Instagram account of a professor at the University of Pennsylvania, where the shooter attended college. Rather, King's philosophy reminds us that courage isn't only about action but about how that action aligns with our values and long-term goals.

Imagination: Envisioning Radical Healthcare Transformation

Imagination in healthcare is often about seeing beyond immediate limitations to create systems that better serve humanity. A compelling example is the transformation of Rwanda's health system after the genocide of the 1990s. Left devastated, Rwanda rebuilt its healthcare infrastructure with an innovative approach that emphasized universal access, community health workers, and public-private partnerships.

By rethinking traditional models, Rwanda achieved remarkable outcomes: reduced child mortality, near-universal health insurance coverage, and significant improvements in life expectancy. This imaginative reengineering of healthcare not only served a struggling nation but became a global model for equitable care in resource-limited settings.

The Will to Rebuild: A Patient's Journey

The will to rebuild can also be intensely personal. Consider David Fajgenbaum, MD, a physician who nearly died five times from Castleman disease, a rare and deadly condition. When traditional treatments failed, he turned his experience into a mission to find answers. Fajgenbaum systematically analyzed his own medical data and repurposed an existing drug to save his life.

His recovery wasn't just a testament to perseverance; it showcased how determination can lead to breakthroughs that benefit others. Fajgenbaum now leads research efforts that are giving hope to patients with rare diseases worldwide. His story illustrates the extraordinary resilience needed to rebuild a life – and, by extension, a path forward for others.

Applying These Lessons Today

In moments of crisis, it is tempting to retreat into cynicism or inaction. But previous challenges remind us that courage, imagination, and the will to rebuild are antidotes to despair.

Today, as we face challenges like climate change, political polarization, and systemic inequality, including in health care, these qualities are more important than ever. Courage is needed to confront powerful interests and demand change. Imagination is required to envision sustainable, equitable systems that serve all people. And the will to rebuild must sustain us through the hard, unglamorous work of implementation and adaptation.

Renewal is possible, but it begins with a decision to reject hopelessness and embrace the possibility of transformation. Just as others have done in the past, we too can rise above malaise to forge a future worthy of our aspirations. But in order to do that, we must overcome our collective anger, unlike Michael Moore, the famous filmmaker, who remarked after the United Healthcare CEO was gunned down: "I'm not going to tamp it [anger] down or ask people to shut up. I want to pour gasoline on that anger."

Many years ago, during my time as a psychiatric resident, I was treating a patient burdened by anger. My supervisor said, "Art, tell your patient that anger is like gasoline: you can light a match to it and make it explosive, or you can put it in your gas tank and get mileage out of it. It depends on how you use it."

I fear that too many of us will want to choose option one and ignore the virtues of option two. But only option two – channeling anger in constructive ways – will build a better America and a stronger healthcare system.

38.

The Season of Hate and Resistance to Healing

The promise of renewal awaits the melting of the ice.

After posting the previous essay online, I was utterly surprised by the hostility it sparked, evident in the overwhelmingly negative comments and the numerous "upvotes" those comments received. Having spent over 40 years as a psychiatric clinician specializing in anger management, I have never encountered such intense anger, ironically directed at its treatment.

One possible explanation can be found in the lyrics of the Pete Seeger 1958 song, "Turn, Turn, Turn," based on the third chapter of Ecclesiastes and popularized by the 1960's rock band, The Byrds. The famous lines are:

> "To every thing, there is a season, and a time to every person under heaven.
> A time to kill, and a time to heal;
> A time to break down and a time to build up;
> A time to love and a time to hate."

> I fear that today is a season of hate. Attempting anger management is like trying to germinate seeds dropped into a cauldron of an erupting volcano.

Although my essay was well-intentioned, it was clearly a non-starter for many people. It got me wondering whether a phase of "pre-contemplation" is necessary before we can be receptive to anger management advice – the same phase considered prerequisite for entering treatment for substance use.

A Season of Hate

There is no doubt that we are living through a "season of hate," where anger has become a default emotional response, amplified by social media, divisive politics, and widespread disillusionment with institutions. Anger, in this context, often functions as a shield – protecting people from vulnerability, sadness, or a sense of powerlessness.

In such an environment, calls for anger management may feel threatening. They are perceived not as tools for empowerment but as demands for self-suppression, particularly if people believe their anger is justified or necessary for survival. Attempting to "germinate seeds" in this volcanic climate may indeed be futile without first addressing the deeper emotional and cognitive state of the audience.

Pre-Contemplation: A Prerequisite for Emotional Growth?

In the stages of change model proposed by the psychologists James O. Prochaska and Carlo C. DiClemente in the late 1970s and early 1980s, pre-contemplation is the stage where individuals are not yet ready to acknowledge their need for change. They may be unaware of the problem, in denial about its impact, or simply resistant to intervention. The model is widely used in various fields, including addiction treatment, health promotion, and psychotherapy, to tailor interventions to an individual's readiness to change.

The stages in the model are:

1. **Pre-contemplation**: No intention to change behavior in the near future.
2. **Contemplation**: Awareness of the need for change and consideration of taking action, but no commitment yet.
3. **Preparation**: Intent to take action soon, often accompanied by small initial steps.
4. **Action**: Active efforts to change behavior.
5. **Maintenance**: Sustained change over time, with a focus on preventing relapse.

It's possible that a similar dynamic applies to anger management. Before people can embrace strategies for managing their anger, they may need to develop awareness of its consequences. Just as individuals with substance use issues often need to see the negative impact of their behavior before contemplating change, those consumed by anger may need to experience its personal costs – alienation, health problems, or unfulfilled goals – before they're open to management techniques.

Equally important is validating their emotions. People may resist anger management advice if they feel their anger is dismissed or delegitimized. Validating the underlying causes of anger – while distinguishing between healthy expression and destructive behavior – could be a crucial step toward engagement. In a climate of widespread mistrust, particularly toward authority figures or perceived elites, building trust is also essential. I would have hoped that my credentials as a psychiatrist would have established credibility, but even then, it seems people may have projected their broader frustrations onto me as the author of the essay.

A Path Forward

If anger management requires a pre-contemplative phase, the question becomes: as therapists, how do we guide people into it? One possible approach is to focus on stories. Narrative medicine teaches us the power of stories to connect emotionally with others. Sharing stories of individuals who have successfully navigated anger and found healing – without instructing or preaching –might help angry people see themselves in those journeys.

It may also help to normalize resistance. Resistance to anger management advice is normal, especially in a culture steeped in anger. This can disarm defensiveness and open the door to reflection. Additionally, offering small wins, such as brief moments of mindfulness or reflective writing, can provide accessible practices that don't feel like full-fledged anger management but can plant the seed of change.

Reframing the message is another critical strategy. The "gasoline" metaphor I described in the previous essay views anger not as suppression but as empowerment – a way to channel anger into effective action and maintain control in a chaotic world. By shifting the narrative, people may come to see these strategies as tools for liberation rather than constraints.

Reflecting on the Response

The backlash to my essay, though painful, is itself a reflection of the very issues I've tried to address. The hostility underscores the urgency of this conversation and the difficulty of engaging with it in a "season of hate." By considering the role of pre-contemplation and exploring alternative ways to reach people, our work as psychotherapists could serve as a bridge to healing in a time when it's needed most.

One of my favorite recording artists, Gil Scott-Heron (1949-2011), penned the song "Winter in America." The lyrics tell of a time when all the seasons were overtaken by the winter, when "all of the healers have been killed or been betrayed…and ain't nobody fighting 'cause nobody knows what to save." This haunting imagery captures the paralysis and despair that can settle in during periods of deep societal or personal unrest.

Yet, even in winter, the earth quietly prepares for spring. Beneath the frozen ground, seeds lie dormant, waiting for warmth and light to awaken them. Perhaps the anger and hostility we see today are the bitter winds of this metaphorical winter, signaling the urgent need for a new season to come.

For that renewal to occur, we must cultivate the conditions for change. We need to thaw the icy grip of cynicism with small acts of kindness, validate anger while guiding it toward constructive action, and, most importantly, nurture the courage and imagination to envision a better future. Winter is not the end; it is a season in transition. As painful as it may be, it holds the possibility of transformation – if we are willing to tend to the seeds of hope and healing.

With patience and determination, we can emerge from this season of anger into a time of rebuilding and renewal, proving that even in the coldest winters, spring will always find its way.

39.

Advancing Innovation Through Responsible Medical Research

Psychedelic drugs are charting a course toward novel therapies while demanding scientific and ethical rigor.

I received a letter from the chairman of a psychiatry department at one of the most highly regarded medical institutions in the world. In the letter, the chairman introduced himself – we do not know one another – and he described the many advanced programs and areas of research in the department. He wrote, "The latest additions to our outpatient offerings [include] the Clinic for Post-Psychedelic Difficulties. This unique clinic offers specialized medical and psychotherapeutic support for people facing challenges of any kind following psychedelic use."

The resurgence of psychedelics in clinical practice marks a significant shift in modern psychiatry and medicine as we begin to explore their therapeutic potential after decades of stigma and prohibition. Historically associated with countercultural movements of the 1960s and recreational use, substances like psilocybin, LSD, and MDMA (ecstasy) are now being rigorously studied for their ability to treat a variety of mental health conditions. This reappraisal stems from an increasing body of evidence demonstrating that psychedelics, when administered in controlled settings with individuals trained as "guides," can produce significant, lasting benefits for patients who have not responded to conventional treatments.

Psychiatry, often at the cutting edge of addressing human suffering, finds itself once again navigating uncharted territory, blending ancient practices and cultural wisdom with modern scientific inquiry. The therapeutic and consciousness-raising potential of psilocybin, in particular, is being vigorously explored at the chairperson's institution.

Research there to date has demonstrated the safety of psilocybin in regulated spaces facilitated by medical teams over a series of guided sessions; and in conjunction with cognitive behavioral therapy, psilocybin has helped reduce anxiety in some cancer patients, and facilitate smoking cessation for others. Additional areas under investigation include PTSD, substance use disorders (opioids, alcohol, and cannabis), anorexia nervosa, treatment-resistant depression, obsessive-compulsive disorder, and post-treatment Lyme disease syndrome (formerly known as chronic Lyme disease).

Yet, as medicine advances, it is essential to acknowledge and prepare for the uncertainties and risks that accompany these breakthroughs. The letter from the chairman highlights this duality. The establishment of the Clinic for Post-Psychedelic Difficulties underscores the need to address the unintended consequences of psychedelics, even as we celebrate their promise. This unique clinic reflects the growing recognition that not all psychedelic experiences are therapeutic, nor are they universally safe. Individuals may encounter psychological distress, exacerbate pre-existing mental health conditions, or struggle with integration – the process of making sense of and applying insights gained during psychedelic experiences.

The re-emergence of psychedelics also raises troubling ethical issues. How do we ensure equitable access to these therapies, particularly when they are restricted (Schedule 1) and may be cost-prohibitive? What safeguards are needed to prevent misuse, over-commercialization, or exploitation within this burgeoning field? How do we prepare clinicians to manage not only the therapeutic administration of psychedelics but also the fallout from unsupervised or improperly conducted experiences? These challenges require a strong framework of education, regulation, and ongoing research to ensure that the promises of psychedelics are not overshadowed by preventable harms. The FDA approval of MDMA-assisted therapy for PTSD, for example, hinges on the manufacturer doing an additional study demonstrating the drug's safety and efficacy. Such studies generally take several years and millions of dollars to conduct.

The broader integration of non-traditional therapies into mainstream medicine is not without precedent. Psychiatry has long been a discipline willing to explore novel interventions, from electroconvulsive therapy to transcranial magnetic stimulation. However, the introduction of psychedelics represents a more pronounced cultural and philosophical shift, one that asks us to reconsider our definitions of healing, consciousness, and even spirituality. In doing so, psychiatry is reclaiming its role as a field that is both deeply scientific and fundamentally humanistic.

For every groundbreaking treatment, there are potential risks and unforeseen effects – a sobering reminder that exploring the frontier of medicine is rarely without peril. Examples from other areas of medicine echo this theme: gene-editing technologies like CRISPR, while revolutionary, raise fears of misuse and unintended genetic consequences; artificial intelligence, a powerful tool in diagnostics, has also been linked to biases and errors that can harm patients.

As psychiatry and medicine continue to embrace the advancements of the "new frontier," it is crucial that we maintain a balanced perspective. Innovation must be tempered with caution, optimism with vigilance. The chairman's initiative to address post-psychedelic challenges exemplifies a responsible approach to progress, one that acknowledges both the potential and the pitfalls of cutting-edge research. Ultimately, the success of these endeavors will depend on our tolerance for risk and ability to ensure that every step forward is guided by compassion, ethics, and an unwavering commitment to the well-being of those we serve.

At the very least, novel clinical research undertaken within any field of medicine requires collaboration with the best multidisciplinary scientists, rigorous basic science research to elucidate underlying mechanisms of action, rigorous clinical trials that adhere to the highest ethical standards, and evidence-based education to clinicians and the broader community to contribute to the development of innovative therapeutic approaches that benefit individuals and society.

40.

Research Misconduct and Questionable Research Practices – Part 1

Conducting unethical research may be tantamount to committing felonies and misdemeanors.

Imagine my surprise in discovering that a few of the articles I had intended to use as research references for essays in this book had been discredited and retracted after they were published in reputable medical journals. Articles that have been retracted from medical journals due to scientific misconduct can be tracked online at Retraction Watch (retractionwatch.com), an organization dedicated to reporting on scientific retractions and related issues. Regrettably, some papers continue to be cited after they have been retracted, as if their research results were still valid.

The Importance of Research Integrity

Research is the bedrock of medical advancement, shaping clinical guidelines, informing public health policies, and guiding patient care. However, the integrity of medical research can be compromised by research misconduct and questionable research practices (QRPs). These unethical behaviors threaten the credibility of findings, jeopardize patient safety, and erode public trust in the medical profession.

Forms of Research Misconduct

Research misconduct often takes the form of fabrication, falsification, or plagiarism. Fabrication involves making up data or results, as seen in the infamous case of Dr. Andrew Wakefield's fraudulent study published in *The Lancet* in 1998 (February 28) linking the MMR vaccine to autism.

This fabricated data contributed to widespread vaccine hesitancy and public health crises.

Falsification refers to manipulating research materials, equipment, or processes to produce a desired outcome, such as selectively cherry-picking data to misrepresent results.

Plagiarism, the unauthorized use or imitation of another researcher's work without proper attribution, undermines academic integrity and disrespects intellectual property. These actions not only compromise the scientific process but also corrode the ethical foundation of medicine.

Questionable Research Practices (QRPs)

Beyond outright misconduct, QRPs present more subtle but pervasive challenges. P-hacking, for instance, involves manipulating data or statistical methods to achieve significant p-values. HARKing – an acronym for "Hypothesizing After the Results are Known" – misleads readers and distorts the scientific record. Other questionable practices include duplicate publication to inflate academic credentials and authorship misconduct, such as including honorary authors who did not contribute to the work or excluding deserving contributors.

Suppressing negative results is another prevalent issue, creating a bias in the literature often referred to as the "file drawer problem." A well-known example of this issue involved the suppression of negative results from clinical trials studying antidepressant medications in children and adolescents. This created a misleading impression of the drug's efficacy and safety, with significant consequences for patient care.

Conflicts of Interest and Ethical Violations

Financial conflicts of interest further complicate research integrity, with studies funded by industry more likely to report positive outcomes, raising concerns about impartiality. Ethical violations, such as conducting studies without informed consent or adequate ethical review, have caused harm, as exemplified by the Tuskegee Syphilis Study. In this infamous case, treatment for syphilis was withheld from African American men without their knowledge to study disease progression, leaving a legacy of mistrust that continues to affect public health efforts.

Prevalence and Systemic Challenges

The distinguished British physician Jeffrey K. Aronson highlights the dangers of research misconduct and QRPs, categorizing them as academic "felonies" and "misdemeanors," respectively. He warns that questionable research practices may drift into outright misconduct. Surveys reveal troubling trends, with approximately 2% of scientists admitting to engaging in fabrication, falsification, or plagiarism, and up to a third admitting to other questionable practices. Reports about colleagues' behavior suggest even higher rates, with up to 14% admitting to falsification and 72% to other QRPs. These behaviors reflect systemic issues such as the pressure to publish, secure funding, and achieve recognition.

Consequences of Research Misconduct

There are major consequences of research misconduct, particularly for patients. Fraudulent findings can lead to harmful or ineffective treatments, exposing patients to unnecessary risks and delaying effective interventions. The Wakefield case, for instance, not only eroded vaccine confidence but also led to outbreaks of preventable diseases like measles. Misconduct tarnishes the reputation of the medical profession, eroding public trust and fostering skepticism about legitimate findings. This distrust can discourage patients from following medical advice or participating in clinical trials, undermining medical progress. Additionally, misconduct wastes financial and human resources, as retractions, investigations, and corrective studies consume funds that could have been directed toward genuine advancements.

Upholding Research Integrity

To address these challenges, the medical community must prioritize education and training in research ethics, ensuring that researchers understand the importance of integrity and the consequences of misconduct. Institutional Review Boards (IRBs) and funding agencies must rigorously evaluate research protocols, while transparency should be promoted through initiatives like mandatory trial registration and open data sharing. Whistleblower protections are crucial, empowering individuals to report misconduct without fear of retaliation. Reforms in publishing, such as stricter peer review processes, mandatory conflict-of-interest disclosures, and adherence to reporting guidelines like CONSORT or PRISMA, can further uphold the quality of research.

Conclusion

Research misconduct and QRPs undermine the foundation of medical progress, posing risks to patient safety and public trust. By acknowledging the prevalence of these issues and implementing universal reforms, the medical community can uphold the highest standards of integrity. Medicine, as both a science and an art, depends on the trust it inspires – a trust that must be safeguarded at all costs.

41.

Research Misconduct and Questionable Research Practices – Part 2

Meting out punishment to fraudsters.

Punishing individuals involved in scientific misconduct and questionable research practices (QRPs) is a delicate matter, as it must balance accountability with the goal of maintaining a fair and productive academic environment. Misconduct and QRPs can have serious consequences, not only for the individuals involved but also for public trust in science and the well-being of patients or society at large. However, any system of punishment must also be equitable, transparent, and focused on prevention, rather than simply retribution.

Formal Sanctions and Retraction of Publications

The most direct consequence of scientific misconduct is the retraction or correction of published papers. Retractions send a clear signal that the work was flawed or fraudulent, and that it can no longer be considered reliable. Retraction, however, is not a substitute for further punitive measures, as its effects on an individual's career can vary greatly depending on their field and reputation. Misconduct-related retractions should be accompanied by formal sanctions such as suspension or termination of the individual's position at an academic institution.

Loss of Funding and Research Opportunities

One of the most impactful consequences of misconduct is the potential loss of research funding. Grant agencies like the National Institutes of Health (NIH) or the National Science Foundation (NSF) often blacklist researchers found guilty of scientific misconduct, preventing them from receiving future funding. This can be devastating to a researcher's career and provides a strong deterrent against unethical behavior.

Furthermore, institutions and research organizations should have mechanisms to bar researchers found guilty of misconduct from supervising students or conducting independent research for a set period, or even indefinitely, depending on the severity of the offense.

Career Consequences

The reputational damage from being found guilty of scientific misconduct can be career-ending. While some researchers may return to the field after a period of reflection, others may find it difficult to rebuild trust within the scientific community. This is a natural consequence of misconduct, as trust is the foundation of scientific collaboration and progress. However, career-ending penalties should be reserved for the most egregious cases of fraud or harm, while lesser infractions (such as some QRPs) might warrant corrective action and education rather than permanent professional exclusion.

Education and Rehabilitation

While punishment is necessary, the scientific community should also consider measures of education and rehabilitation for those who engage in less severe forms of misconduct or QRPs. These individuals may benefit from training on research ethics, best practices for data collection and analysis, and the importance of transparency. Providing opportunities for researchers to correct their mistakes and re-enter the scientific community under new ethical guidelines can help foster a culture of integrity.

For minor QRPs, such as selective reporting or p-hacking, education on proper statistical methods and the importance of transparency may suffice to correct behavior. It's important to view these individuals as having made a mistake that can be addressed, rather than irreparably damaging their careers.

Public Disclosures and Accountability

Transparency is crucial in dealing with scientific misconduct. Institutions, journals, and funding agencies should have clear procedures for investigating allegations of misconduct and should ensure that these investigations are impartial and thorough. Publicly disclosing the results of investigations and the sanctions applied can act as a deterrent for others and help maintain the public's trust in science. However, this must be done carefully to avoid unjustly ruining careers over unfounded allegations or minor infractions.

Public Apology

It's uncommon for those who perpetrate scientific fraud it to come forward. However, there are exceptions. Recently, a scientist who worked at a Philadelphia, Pennsylvania children's hospital and later a biotechnology company admitted to falsifying data in cardiovascular research, leading to the retraction of two of her papers. In a highly unusual confession, the researcher admitted to manipulating samples and incorrectly reporting data to achieve the desired result. The other authors of the paper were unaware of the misconduct, yet they were forced to share the blame, writing: "[We] would like to sincerely apologize to the members of staff of [the journal], the reviewers who provided the reviews for the manuscript, and all who were involved in the publication of this manuscript and anyone who is impacted by the actions of the [guilty individual]."

Collaborative Accountability and Peer Review

Institutions, journals, and research collaborators should work together to ensure that research is conducted ethically and to hold individuals accountable when misconduct occurs. This collaborative approach is key to identifying QRPs early in the process, reducing the likelihood of widespread damage to scientific literature.

Peer reviewers also play a critical role in preventing misconduct by identifying potential red flags in submitted manuscripts and flagging issues like data inconsistencies, lack of transparency, or missing ethical approvals.

In one incident, researchers attempted to determine the prevalence of unprofessional social media content among vascular surgery residents. The researchers accessed the residents' Facebook, Twitter, and Instagram accounts without permission, resulting in a severe backlash from the medical community and an apology from the authors and journal editors for their ethical miscue in not seeking the permission of the residents to use their personally identifying information, as well as other problems with the methodology "in which significant conscious and unconscious biases were pervasive," while also citing "failures in the Journal's peer review process..."

Severity Based on Impact

Not all misconduct or QRPs are equal, and penalties should be proportionate to the severity of the offense. A researcher who falsifies data in a clinical trial that harms patients should face more serious consequences, including potential legal action and permanent expulsion from the field, compared to a researcher who inadvertently fails to disclose a minor conflict of interest. Misconduct that directly threatens public health or safety should be met with the most severe penalties.

For minor infractions – such as improper citation or poor data handling –remedial actions like formal warnings, additional training, or publication corrections may suffice. However, when misconduct endangers public trust, patient care, or the integrity of scientific fields, the penalties should be stricter.

Conclusion

I'm reminded of *The Fugitive,* the 1993 film starring Harrison Ford as Dr. Richard Kimble, a prominent Chicago vascular surgeon wrongfully convicted of murdering his wife. A key subplot involves research misconduct, as Kimble uncovers a conspiracy related to a pharmaceutical company's fraudulent activities. A compromised pathologist working for the company falsifies research data to gain approval for a new drug, leading to severe surgical complications from excessive bleeding. Although the pathologist, Dr. Charles Nichols (played by Jeroen Krabbé), is apprehended, we never do learn his fate.

Forgetting for the moment that Dr. Nichols was complicit in the death of Dr. Kimble's wife, what punishment would you suggest for his falsifying the research data?

42.

Consequences of the FDA's Purge of Website Diversity Content

New federal policies fundamentally alter how researchers and companies approach drug and medical device testing.

The Trump administration's directive to eliminate diversity, equity, and inclusion (DEI) language and initiatives from federal government agencies has had significant consequences, particularly within the Food and Drug Administration (FDA). The removal of DEI-related content from the FDA's website, including resources that promote diversity in clinical trials, highlights broader implications for healthcare policy, drug development, and public trust in the medical system.

Efforts to enhance diversity in clinical trials have been recognized as vital to ensuring that experimental drugs and devices are tested across varied populations that represent the broader patient demographics they are intended to serve. Diversity in clinical trials not only improves scientific validity but also addresses disparities in healthcare outcomes.

Historically, a lack of representation in trials has led to skepticism among underrepresented groups and gaps in understanding how certain treatments affect diverse populations. For example, early trials of cholesterol-lowering drugs primarily enrolled men, leaving questions about their efficacy in women unanswered until later studies demonstrated their life-saving benefits. Similarly, certain medications, such as hydralazine/isosorbide for heart failure, have been approved specifically for African Americans, and cancer drugs targeting genes more common in Asian populations underscore the necessity of inclusive research.

The FDA, under the Biden administration, sought to address these disparities by urging industry stakeholders to enroll more women and people of color in trials, issuing draft guidance in 2024 to this effect (now deleted). However, the Trump administration's removal of such guidance and other DEI-related resources introduces uncertainty into the regulatory framework, potentially stalling progress in creating equitable healthcare solutions. The lack of clear directives risks undermining years of advocacy and progress toward inclusive clinical research.

The removal of DEI content extends beyond the FDA. Pages from agencies like the National Cancer Institute and the National Institutes of Health (NIH) have also been deleted, including those supporting research on sexual and gender minority health and women's health. This sweeping policy shift reflects a broader governmental retreat from DEI principles, which could have cascading effects on research priorities and public health initiatives.

The implications of these actions are far-reaching. Without institutional support for diversity in research, clinical trials may revert to outdated practices, perpetuating systemic biases in drug development. For pharmaceutical companies and researchers, the absence of clear federal guidance may create operational challenges and lead to inconsistent adherence to best practices in patient recruitment. For patients, especially those from marginalized communities, diminished representation in trials could exacerbate healthcare inequities and erode trust in medical interventions.

Moreover, the administration's directives have disrupted the FDA's operations, as staff members grapple with identifying which programs are considered DEI-related and therefore subject to termination. The lack of clarity and sudden removal of resources have created an environment of confusion and apprehension within the agency. These disruptions threaten to impact critical functions, including advisory committee meetings crucial for drug approval processes and communication with stakeholders, potentially delaying the drug approval process.

The unease within the FDA and other health agencies is palpable, as staff navigate the ambiguity of what constitutes a DEI program. The administration's directive has led to the termination of DEI offices and contracts, and employees have been instructed to report any attempts to maintain DEI efforts covertly. This environment of uncertainty is compounded by restrictions on travel and communication, which could impact the FDA's operational effectiveness. Plus, many of Trump's executive orders are in legal limbo as attorney general representing many states, and other stakeholders, argue their legalities.

The broader policy implications of these actions also touch on fundamental questions about the role of government in regulating healthcare and scientific research, as discussed in essay 32. By prioritizing political ideologies over evidence-based practices, the administration risks compromising the integrity of medical research and undermining public confidence in regulatory institutions. Furthermore, the executive order's call to report "coded or imprecise language" used to disguise DEI programs fosters an atmosphere of surveillance and fear, which could discourage innovative approaches to addressing health disparities.

In summary, the removal of DEI-related resources from federal agencies like the FDA underscores the dangers of political interference in healthcare policy. Diversity in clinical trials is not merely a matter of fairness but a scientific necessity to ensure treatments are safe and effective for all populations. The far-reaching implications of these policy changes extend beyond the immediate disruption of clinical research, threatening to deepen healthcare inequities and compromise the credibility of regulatory agencies. Policymakers must carefully consider the long-term consequences of prioritizing political agendas over the advancement of equitable and evidence-based medical practices.

43.

Citizenship Should Not Be a Condition of Treatment

The Hippocratic Oath does not make a distinction.

The Hippocratic Oath does not require citizenship as a condition of treatment. The Oath, which serves as a foundational ethical guideline for physicians, emphasizes principles such as doing no harm, maintaining patient confidentiality, and practicing medicine ethically and with integrity. It focuses on the physician's responsibilities to patients and the ethical practice of medicine, rather than any conditions related to a patient's citizenship or nationality.

So, why did this issue surface when a treatment team could not ascertain a patient's citizenship status – his "green card" had expired – and hesitated to treat him? In my 40-plus years of practice, I have never encountered this as a problem, and I've treated many undocumented individuals.

Straying into unfamiliar territory, I decided to research this topic further. I discovered that it is not uncommon for issues related to a patient's citizenship or immigration status to arise in healthcare settings due to administrative and legal considerations rather than medical ethics. One of the main reasons is related to insurance and payment. A patient's citizenship or immigration status can influence their eligibility for certain types of health insurance or public benefits, which can affect their ability to pay for services and present administrative challenges for the treatment team.

Furthermore, healthcare facilities are required to comply with various state and federal regulations. Some of these regulations may necessitate verification of identity and legal status for certain types of care or services.

Additionally, some services, particularly those funded by government programs, may require legal residency or citizenship status for eligibility. Lastly, maintaining accurate patient records is a crucial part of both medical and administrative processes, and uncertainty about a patient's legal status can add a layer of complexity to clinical documentation.

Despite these concerns, it is important to note that the ethical obligation of healthcare providers, as outlined by the Hippocratic Oath and other ethical tenets, is to provide care to all patients regardless of their citizenship status. Therefore, healthcare providers must ensure that these administrative hurdles do not obstruct access to necessary medical care.

Will that still be the case under the Trump administration?

President Trump has implemented numerous immigration policy changes aimed at restricting entry at the border and increasing interior enforcement, including rescinding protections for sensitive areas like schools and healthcare facilities. These measures primarily target undocumented immigrants but have widespread effects on mixed-status families, including U.S.-born children. Enhanced enforcement, including raids and mass deportations, has raised fears among immigrant communities, potentially affecting their health, well-being, employment, and daily life.

Restrictive policies have led to increased stress and anxiety, particularly among children, and deterred immigrant families from accessing health care and social services. Family separations and detentions can result in long-term mental and physical health consequences. Detention facilities are already strained, with reports of poor conditions and inadequate medical care.

When an undocumented individual shows up at your healthcare doorstep, what will you do? The answer, of course, is: treat them. But soon, afterward, you may find ICE agents knocking on that door requesting information about them, including protected health information (PHI), and may even seek to question or detain patients when they have been admitted to the hospital or come to a clinic to obtain treatment, or about visitors to the facility. What is your course of action then?

According to one law firm, to prepare for potential ICE enforcement, healthcare providers should update policies, designate a legal point of contact, train staff on handling law enforcement inquiries, and establish protocols to verify agents' authority. Staff should avoid sharing patient information without legal review, as HIPAA does not require disclosure of PHI except in limited circumstances. Healthcare facilities must balance patient privacy protections with legal obligations while ensuring compliance with law enforcement procedures.

No doubt physicians and other healthcare practitioners will be caught in the crosshairs. Once again, I strongly encourage doctors to provide treatment to undocumented immigrants. Providing therapy is firmly in keeping with The Hippocratic Oath and medical ethics that support treating all patients without discrimination. We went to medical school to learn how to provide care based on medical need, not legal status. Besides, ensuring access to health care for everyone, including undocumented immigrants, helps prevent the spread of infectious diseases, reduces emergency room overcrowding, and improves overall community health.

And let's not forget that in the U.S., federal law, specifically the Emergency Medical Treatment and Labor Act (EMTALA), requires hospitals to provide emergency care to all individuals, regardless of immigration status or ability to pay. Many undocumented immigrants face significant barriers to accessing care, leading to untreated chronic conditions, poor health outcomes, and higher long-term health costs. Providing care aligns with principles of compassion and justice.

While some argue that treating undocumented migrants strains health care resources, research suggests that they contribute to the economy through taxes and labor. Additionally, preventive and routine care can reduce costly emergency interventions. Ultimately, doctors should focus on their role as healers, advocating for equitable healthcare access while leaving administrators to deal with laws and institutional policies.

44.

Don't Dream It's Over – Yet

The epidemic of global violence can be addressed through personal conviction and government coordination.

Many songs and famous refrains flooded my mind as we transitioned into 2025, where domestic and international strife dotted the landscape. "Living on a thin line," "It all over now baby blue," and "Can't find my way home," were some of the notable downers. On the flip side (no pun intended), I was uplifted by "Land of hope and dreams" and "It's gonna be a bright sun-shiny day," as well as the belief that "Love reign o'er me."

Of all, what stood out was "Don't Dream It's Over," a hit song written in 1986 by New Zealand-born Neil Finn. It is the most well-known song by his group, Crowded House, and an anthem for many. Finn reflects, "I was contemplating the end of things: relationships and the challenges that you face. It's an exhortation to myself – and to anyone who's going through that – to not think it's the end, to keep on pushing, keep on believing. It's a song of hope, I think."

Yet, like many of Finn's songs, there are also strains of melancholia, even hopelessness – for example, the line "In the paper today tales of war and of waste, but you turn right over to the T.V. page." Have we really become so numb to violence that our only solution is to ignore it? Are we helpless to solve the epidemic of violence in America and elsewhere, consigned to simply watching it repeatedly unfold – on television and in the newspaper – and flipping a switch or turning the page in resignation?

Finn said that, in a sense, "Don't Dream It's Over" was a "private message…to someone who was withdrawing from their world." In an era now dominated by war and where mass casualty incidents are commonplace – whether at a German Christmas market or on New Year's Day in New Orleans – withdrawal is the last thing we should do.

The temptation to disengage, to retreat from the onslaught of despair that headlines bring, is understandable. Yet, if we withdraw, who will be left to advocate for change? The world does not heal itself passively; it requires action, hope, and effort. Finn's refrain – "They come to build a wall between us; don't ever let them win" – reminds us to "keep pushing, keep believing," even when the odds seem insurmountable.

Governments and countries have the power to tackle the widespread violence through deliberate and coordinated strategies. First, addressing the root causes of violence – such as poverty, inequality, and lack of education – can reduce the desperation and resentment that often lead to conflict. Investing in social safety nets, job creation, and equitable economic policies can provide alternatives to violence and foster stability.

Second, international cooperation is vital. Institutions like the United Nations must be strengthened – not weakened – to mediate disputes, prevent conflicts, and hold accountable those who perpetuate violence. Diplomatic engagement, peacekeeping missions, and arms control agreements are tools that can curb large-scale violence. Additionally, enforcing stricter regulations on the global arms trade can help limit the availability of weapons in volatile regions.

Third, education and community programs that promote tolerance and understanding can undermine the narratives of hate and division that fuel violence. Governments can support initiatives that counter extremist ideologies, empower marginalized communities, and promote peaceful conflict resolution.

Finally, addressing the role of the media is essential. While free speech is a cornerstone of democracy, sensationalized coverage of violence can desensitize audiences or amplify fear. Governments and media organizations must work together to promote responsible reporting that informs without inciting.

Perhaps this is where Finn's message becomes truly universal: hope and despair are not mutually exclusive. The act of dreaming, of striving for better, can coexist with the acknowledgment of difficulty and pain. It is this tension that gives the song its emotional resonance and makes it enduringly relevant.

In a modern context, “Don’t Dream It’s Over” is not just a statement of personal resilience; it’s a call to collective action. It challenges us to look at the tales of war and waste and not turn away in apathy. Instead, it dares us to envision solutions, to rebuild broken systems, and to nurture a world where hope is not a fleeting sentiment but a sustainable reality.

While it’s easy to feel overwhelmed by the enormity of the world’s problems, Finn’s lyrics whisper a quieter truth: each of us has a role to play. Small acts of courage, kindness, and advocacy can ripple outward, creating change in ways we may never fully see or understand.

So, let us take to heart Finn’s exhortation. The challenges we face, though daunting, can be overcome. Don’t dream it’s over. Because as long as there are people willing to dream, to hope, and to act, there is always a chance for something better.

And to all who respond negatively to this essay, “you’ll never see the end of the road while you’re travelling with me.”

Afterword

45.

The Limits of Medicine and New Frontiers

As I remarked in the Prologue – and despite the somewhat downbeat tone of many of these essays – I remain optimistic about the overall future of American medicine. But optimism does not erase the challenges we face or the limitations inherent to our efforts. These hurdles shape our journey and test our resolve.

The concept of new frontiers and the multiverse was vividly illustrated in an episode of *Star Trek* (the original television series) titled "The City on the Edge of Forever." In this classic story, Joan Collins portrays Edith Keeler, an idealistic social worker devoted to uplifting humanity during the Great Depression.

In this memorable episode, often regarded as *Star Trek's* finest, Kirk and Spock find themselves in 1930s Earth, seeking Dr. McCoy, who, in a delusional state, has accidentally transported himself to that era. Kirk and Spock do not know exactly when or where they will intersect with McCoy, heightening the tension of their mission.

Spock explains to Kirk – who is falling in love with Keeler – that two potential futures hinge on her fate. The two possible outcomes are:

1. **Edith Keeler Lives**: If Edith Keeler survives, she goes on to lead a pacifist movement in the United States. Her influence delays the United States' entry into World War II, allowing Nazi Germany to develop the atomic bomb first and ultimately win the war. This outcome results in a drastically altered future where the Federation and Starfleet do not exist.

2. **Edith Keeler Dies**: If Edith Keeler dies, the timeline remains unchanged. The United States enters World War II at the appropriate time, contributing to the eventual Allied victory. This

> ensures that history proceeds as it should, leading to the future where the Federation and Starfleet exist.

The deciding factor, the "random element," is Dr. McCoy.

Spoiler alert: the second scenario proves true. In a poignant moment, Kirk must restrain McCoy from saving Keeler from an oncoming car. Her tragic death ensures that history proceeds as it should, and one of the most romantic episodes in the Star Trek fleet comes to an end.

The parallels to medical practice are striking. Kirk's deliberate inaction, his choice not to save Edith by restraining McCoy, who instinctively moves toward her, illustrates the weight of responsibility and the often-painful nature of medical decision-making. The narrative evokes "The Serenity Prayer," typically recited in Alcoholics Anonymous meetings: "God grant me the serenity to accept the things I cannot change; courage to change the things I can; and wisdom to know the difference…"

In mental health care, I often encounter the tension between idealism and realism. Social workers like Edith Keeler, for instance, advocate for boundless hope and universal redemption. But the constraints of medicine force hard truths: not every patient can be saved. Some will remain chronically ill, others will resist treatment, and still others will refuse help despite their suffering. Resources are finite, and so is our ability to intervene.

We live in a multiverse of infinite possibilities but finite frontiers. When we reach the limits of what we can do, we must make the difficult decision to move on, focusing our energy on those who can benefit most. Is this pragmatism or callousness? Perhaps it is neither – or both. The question itself underscores the delicate balance we must maintain.

Medicine itself is an inflection point. The tension between the idealistic and the pragmatic defines our work as healers. The social worker's unyielding optimism and the physician's tempered realism are not opposing forces but complementary strengths. Without dreamers, we risk stagnation; without realists, we risk ruin.

This dynamic balance drives us toward medicine's new frontiers. As we contend with the limitations of our current knowledge and resources, we must also embrace emerging possibilities. Precision medicine offers hope for individualized care. Artificial intelligence holds the promise of enhancing diagnostics and treatment. Global health initiatives remind us that our frontiers extend beyond borders. Yet, these advancements bring new challenges, including ethical dilemmas, inequities, and unintended consequences – the "random elements" that shape the trajectory of progress.

The lesson of Edith Keeler and "The City on the Edge of Forever" is not to abandon hope or be immobilized by the weight of difficult decisions. Rather, it is to act with intention, guided by wisdom and balanced by both science and compassion. Medicine's frontiers are not fixed destinations but evolving pathways in the multiverse. As caregivers, we journey together, finding meaning not only in what we achieve but in how we navigate the uncertainties and possibilities ahead.

Notes and Sources

Essay 1
1. *Jama Network Open* article: https://jamanetwork.com/journals/jamanetworkopen/fullarticle/2825349.
2. *Advances in Therapy* review article: https://link.springer.com/article/10.1007/s12325-022-02153-x.
3. John F. Kennedy presidential speech remarks: https://archive.org/details/unfinishedlifejo00dall_0/page/275/mode/2up.

Essay 2
1. "What is the Fencing Response?" https://www.verywellhealth.com/fencing-response-7375004.
2. "Bread and Circuses: Ancient Rome, Modern Science Fiction, and the Art of Political Distraction.": https://muse.jhu.edu/article/842291.

Essay 6
1. "A Thin Shred of My Sanity Remained. Then I Hit My Breaking Point," by Dr. Sarah DeParis: https://www.medpagetoday.com/opinion/second-opinions/113489.

Essay 8
1. "Changes coming to weight loss drug coverage benefits, effective January 1, 2025," Independence Blue Cross: https://provcomm.ibx.com/pnc-ibc/news/Pages/Changes-coming-to-weight-loss-drug-coverage-benefits.aspx.
2. The Hartmann Report: https://hartmannreport.com/p/were-it-not-for-white-supremacy-america-d21.
3. *JAMA* article: https://jamanetwork.com/journals/jama/fullarticle/2649174?utm_source=chatgpt.com.
4. *JAMA* editorial by physician researchers: https://jamanetwork.com/journals/jama/fullarticle/2649162.

Essay 11

1. Survey results: https://talkerresearch.com/was-2024-the-worst-year-ever-americans-rate-it-six-out-of-10/.

Essay 13

1. Why doctors marry doctors: Exploring medical marriages: https://www.ama-assn.org/medical-residents/medical-resident-wellness/why-doctors-marry-doctors-exploring-medical-marriages

Essay 14

1. "Testing and Evaluation of Health Applications of Large Language Models: A Systematic Review": https://jamanetwork.com/journals/jama/fullarticle/2825147.

Essay 15

1. Sam Jacobs quote: https://www.magzter.com/stories/News/Time/Time-Person-of-the-Year-Taylor-Swift?srsltid=AfmBOoqdFktvy4_2mHzTKpNUKmkkdrHi56y1UrQM5pSkbGW-OHupqqQV.
2. "Can AI replace psychotherapists? Exploring the future of mental health care.": https://www.frontiersin.org/journals/psychiatry/articles/10.3389/fpsyt.2024.1444382/full.

Essay 19

1. "Age against the machine—susceptibility of large language models to cognitive impairment: cross sectional analysis.": https://www.bmj.com/content/387/bmj-2024-081948.
2. "How spatial abilities enhance, and are enhanced by, dental education.": https://www.sciencedirect.com/science/article/pii/S1041608008000289?via%3Dihub.
3. "Recent evidence on visual-spatial ability in surgical education: A scoping review.": https://pmc.ncbi.nlm.nih.gov/articles/PMC7749687/.

Essay 22

1. "Governing AI for Humanity," United Nations: https://www.un.org/sites/un2.un.org/files/governing_ai_for_humanity_final_report_en.pdf.

Essay 27
1. "Mirror, Mirror 2024: A Portrait of the Failing U.S. Health System: Comparing Performance in 10 Nations": https://www.commonwealthfund.org/publications/fund-reports/2024/sep/mirror-mirror-2024?utm_campaign=Saturday%20Digest&utm_medium=email&_hsenc=p2ANqtz-9v-17qWdw4hTmE4RBj3aecNSU3aZoUxcCy5BWZWDa7gC6TmciHpTTs0tJw5diGu3xRp-5kDWwP7GFVAFwplMziTe2yFw&_hsmi=2&utm_content=2&utm_source=hs_email.
2. "Health Care Administrative Costs in the United States and Canada, 2017": https://www.acpjournals.org/doi/10.7326/M19-2818.

Essay 28
1. Senator Rand Paul quote: https://x.com/RandPaul/status/1881328949021573590?mx=2.

Essay 30
1. "Analysis Predicts Big Drop for U.S. in Global Health Rankings.": https://www.healthday.com/health-news/general-health/analysis-predicts-big-drop-for-us-in-global-health-rankings.
2. *The Lancet* commentary: https://www.thelancet.com/journals/lancet/article/PIIS0140-6736(24)02664-3/fulltext.
3. "Health and Freedom," by Timothy Snyder: https://www.thelancet.com/journals/lancet/article/PIIS0140-6736(24)02664-3/fulltext.

Essay 31
1. AAMC. "New AAMC Data on Medical School Applicants and Enrollment in 2024." https://www.aamc.org/news/press-releases/new-aamc-data-medical-school-applicants-and-enrollment-2024.

Essay 32
1. Teaching Health Center Graduate Medical Education: https://www.thcgme.org/.
2. Physician Pathway Act: https://www.thcgme.org/.

Essay 35
1. Elon Musk tweet: https://www.theguardian.com/world/2024/dec/20/elon-musk-claims-only-afd-can-save-germany.
2. “German far-right AfD in disarray after Nazi remark.”: https://www.bbc.com/news/articles/cx88nwy934go.\

Essay 36
1. Bruce Springsteen quote: https://www.nytimes.com/1992/08/09/arts/pop-music-when-the-boss-fell-to-earth-he-hit-paradise.html.

Essay 37
1. “My Last Column: Finding Hope in an Age of Resentment,” by Paul Krugman: https://www.nytimes.com/2024/12/09/opinion/elites-euro-social-media.html.
2. “Penn condemns professor’s support for alumnus charged with killing CEO.”: https://www.thedp.com/article/2024/12/penn-condemns-professor-comment-luigi-mangione.
3. “A Manifesto Against For-Profit Health Insurance Companies,” by Michael Moore: https://www.michaelmoore.com/p/a-manifesto-against-for-profit-health?utm_medium=web.

Essay 40
1. “When I use a word . . . Academic integrity—defining misdemeanors,” by Jeffrey K. Aronson: https://www.bmj.com/content/387/bmj.q2817.
2. “How Many Scientists Fabricate and Falsify Research? A Systematic Review and Meta-Analysis of Survey Data?”: https://journals.plos.org/plosone/article?id=10.1371/journal.pone.0005738.

Essay 41
1. Retraction notice, *JVS Vas Sci*: https://pmc.ncbi.nlm.nih.gov/articles/PMC11563159/.
2. Retraction notice, *JVS*: https://www.jvascsurg.org/article/S0741-5214(20)31848-6/fulltext.

Essay 43

1. "The Trump Administration's Immigration Enforcement Policy: What Hospitals and Health Care Providers Must Know for Their Patients, Staff, and Visitors": https://www.ebglaw.com/insights/publications/the-trump-administrations-immigration-enforcement-policy-what-hospitals-and-health-care-providers-must-know-for-their-patients-staff-and-visitors.
2. "Who Are the 1 Million Missing Workers that Could Solve America's Labor Shortages?": https://www.brookings.edu/articles/who-are-the-1-million-missing-workers-that-could-solve-americas-labor-shortages/.

Essay 44

1. Neil Finn reflects on "Don't Dream It's Over: https://www.bbc.com/news/articles/cx88nwy934go.
2. Neil Finn quote: https://www.neilfinn.com/dont-dream-its-over.

About the Author

Arthur Lazarus, MD, MBA, is a healthcare consultant, certified physician executive, and nationally recognized author, speaker, and champion of physician leadership and wellness. He has broad experience in clinical practice and the health insurance industry, having led programs at Cigna and Humana. At Humana, Lazarus was vice president and corporate medical director of behavioral health operations in Louisville, Kentucky, and subsequently a population health medical director in the state of Florida.

Lazarus has also held leadership positions in several pharmaceutical companies, including Pfizer and AstraZeneca, conducting clinical trials, and reviewing promotional material for medical accuracy and FDA compliance. He has published more than 450 articles and essays online and in scientific and professional journals and has written and edited over a dozen books, including many related to the field of narrative medicine.

Born in Philadelphia, Pennsylvania, Lazarus attended Boston University, where he graduated with a bachelor's degree in psychology with Distinction. He received his medical degree with Honors from Temple University School of Medicine, followed by a psychiatric residency at Temple University Hospital, where he was chief resident. After residency, Lazarus joined the faculty of Temple University School of Medicine, where he currently serves as Adjunct Professor of Psychiatry. He also holds non-faculty appointments as Executive-in-Residence at Temple University Fox School of Business and Management, where he received his MBA degree, and Senior Fellow, Jefferson College of Population Health, Philadelphia, Pennsylvania.

Well known for his leadership and medical management skills, Lazarus is a sought-after presenter, mentor, teacher, and writer. He has shared his expertise and perspective at numerous local, national, and international meetings and seminars.

Lazarus is a past president of the American Association for Psychiatric Administration and Leadership, a former member of the board of directors of the American Association for Physician Leadership (AAPL), and a current member of the AAPL editorial review board. In 2010, the American Psychiatric Association honored Lazarus with the Administrative Psychiatry Award for his effectiveness as an administrator of major mental health programs and expanding the body of knowledge of management science in mental health services delivery systems.

Lazarus is among a select group of physicians in the United States who have been inducted into both the Alpha Omega Alpha medical honor society and the Beta Gamma Sigma honor society of collegiate schools of business.

Lazarus enjoys walking, biking, playing piano, and listening to music. He has been happily married to his wife, Cheryl, for over 40 years. They are the proud parents of four adult children and the grandparents of six young children.

www.ingramcontent.com/pod-product-compliance
Lightning Source LLC
LaVergne TN
LVHW010718210926
848485LV00008B/1446/J
* 9 7 8 1 6 8 0 5 3 4 0 4 7 *